"As a travel writer, this j

only tells, took me on a

reflect on my own experiences of loss, soothing those memories. I could not put the book down."

—Karen Berger, New York Times bestselling author,
America Great Hiking Trails

"From the opening chapter of this beautiful story, I was invited into the heart of a friendship and the memories of an incredible woman. This memoir reads like a novel and takes the reader on a journey through the intertwined lives of two strong, funny, unapologetic, and colourful women as they navigate love and loss, strengthen their friendship over distance and time, and learn how to let go and say goodbye. This book will make you laugh and cry and will serve as a reminder of the precious nature of life."

—Kate Gajdosik, Producer, IMDb

"A compelling story that leads the reader into the warp and weft of the timeless meaning of friendship between two women. Time can heal, sometimes in unexpected ways."

—Laila Radage, co-author, Through the Golden Age

"As long-time supporters of the Pancreatic Cancer Action Network (PanCAN), and grant donors to help advance research in precision medicine for better treatment of pancreatic cancer, this book eloquently informs of the reality of patients and their families after diagnosis. It also highlights the difficulty of such an emotional journey without the support of an organization such as PanCAN. More than that, it is the captivating story of a friendship."

—Steve, and Cheryl Kole
PanCAN PurpleStride Silicon Valley/
Promise & Progress Team Captain

Biography of A Friendship

Biography of A Friendship

Marie-Claude Arnott

Biography of A Friendship

Tule Publishing First Printing, March 2024

The Tule Publishing, Inc.

First Publication by Tule Publishing 2024

Cover design by Lynn Andreozzi
Author Photo credit: Cindy Dumollard

This book is a memoir. It reflects the author's present recollections of experiences over time. Some names and characteristics have been changed, some events have been compressed, and any dialogue has been recreated to the best of author's memory.

ISBN: 978-1-962707-68-8

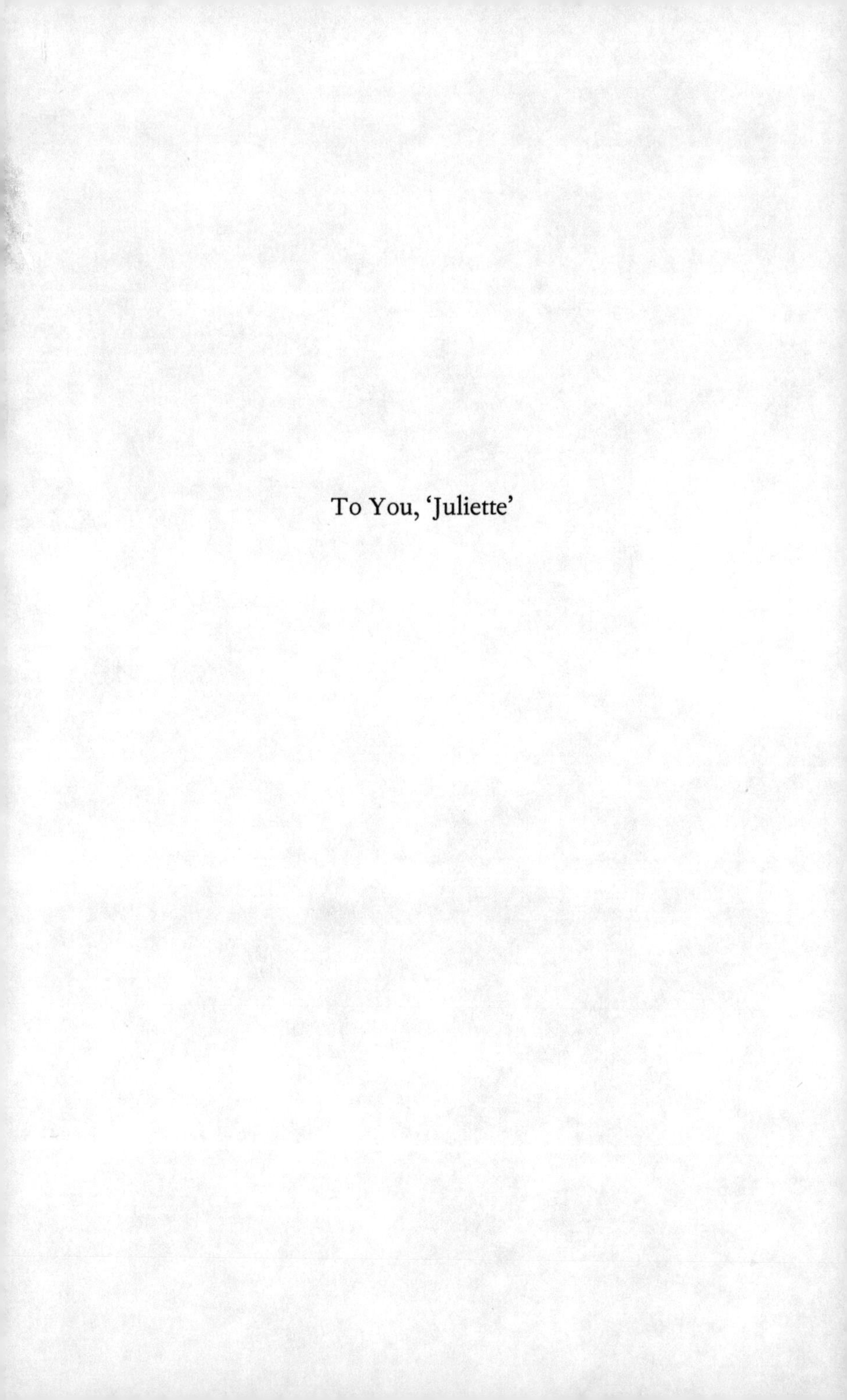

To You, 'Juliette'

TABLE OF CONTENTS

AUTHOR'S NOTE

THIS IS A memoir. I share a personal story to the best of my recollection. At the request of my friend's daughter, the family's real names have been changed. Using real names can feel like an invasion of privacy and goodwill could later become regrets. For this reason, *Marianne* and *Jean-Paul* are fictitious names too. A few inconsequential facts were also changed to protect that privacy. However, none of this affects the core of the story.

Other than a few unforgettable one-liners, the dialogues are a work of creative nonfiction, in the spirit of what was said at the time. The reader gets acquainted with my friend's voice in the colloquial way that best suits her character.

The places I describe are real and in sync with what happened at that narrative moment.

In this story of a friendship affected by an illness, I weave in basic information about pancreatic cancer, as the facts were at the time of printing. I hope this doesn't burden the reader but informs about that silent illness instead.

To facilitate requesting 'permission to use' quotes and material, I chose the Pancreatic Cancer Action Network (PanCAN) as my main source of information, via its comprehensive, user-friendly website.

The use of ellipses in the dialogues indicates a labored speech, a hesitation, or a pause. In the emails, in English or translated from French, the ellipses in brackets […] indicate a text omission, a correction, or an adjustment for relevance or better comprehension.

For a visual experience of the geographical settings in the book, stay tuned to social media.

IN THE WAY OF A COMMENCEMENT

After one of her typical bouts of wit one day, I told my friend I would write a book about her life. I wanted to give her one last gift. A glimpse of a future she would never know. Thirty years of friendship flashed through my mind from the first to the last chapter. At the time, I imagined a biographical novel, recounting our friendship through her colorful life while bearing witness to her short-lived illness. After all, as a freelance writer, I would know how to do this.

Or so I thought.

I couldn't relive my friend's ordeal even as the heroine of a fictionalized story. That our friendship and my friend had become a memory confused me. It was like looking from my window at the fog over the Pacific Ocean of the Northwest and having to imagine the water.

Eight months passed before I could write the first sentence of the first paragraph. Serendipity had me stumble upon NaNoWriMo—the National Novel Writing Month: writers pledge to write a 50,000-word novel during November only.

All I had to do was begin to write and keep writing an average of 1,666 words per day for thirty days. I felt like I had been swallowed by a wave and had to swim or sink. The challenge dragged untapped thoughts from my mind, my fingers rushing on the keyboard often through the night.

When my submission was finally validated, I had completed the first draft—no duplication of chapters or paragraphs, no plagiarism, and the requested word count. Relief was short-lived as doubts snuck in before I began the second draft. I was experiencing first-hand why it's so difficult to write a book. What's more, about a loss.

I had raced through the first draft but would have to relive it slowly and intently, prodding my memories to develop it. Sharing my friend's complicated life through our friendship was one thing, but writing about her illness was another: I felt like I would have to make her die 'again.'

More complicated was exposing her private life, not that she ever told me what I could and couldn't write. Still, I got so entangled with issues of ethics and loyalty that I was losing my sense of purpose. My friend's legacy would be a forgotten manuscript found someday in some boxes…

Then, one thing led to another.

I was working on a writing tutorial by Susan Tiberghien and identified with her life stories. And as serendipity would again have it, she lives in Switzerland, yet close to my family in France. We ended up meeting in a café in Geneva, and our conversation quickly turned to my so-called *biographical novel.*

"It's not a biographical novel!" she said with the vivacity of someone who knows for sure. "It's a memoir!" As a memoirist, she knew: "It's *your* experience of *your* friendship along with *your* recollection of *your* friend's life by way of her terminal illness."

Unlike a novel, a memoir is about facts and is written in the first person. I just had to tell the story as it happened. It didn't make the process easier, but it gave me a clearer course of action and a renewed sense of purpose. Still, I often had to step back or pause to get perspective.

Writing a memoir takes you on a convoluted journey, unexpected for sure as it keeps pulling gems from your psyche. It can't be rushed and only *you* will know when your story has completed its arc. You will know because it won't leave you alone until you reach its cathartic meaning. And from this, an enlightened *you* will rise.

CHAPTER 1

California, February 2014

I LOOK OUT the window as if it were the last time and see it for the first time. Nature plays with my mind even from the sofa where I lie. I don't hear the chirping of the sparrows sipping in the fountain, but I hear it in my head, and the hummingbird fluttering over a salvia bloom reminds me that blooming perennials always linger through California's mild winters. Even the garden is in transition, neither dormant nor growing.

I ponder the dualities in life and its conundrums. I take in details, as in *before it might be too late*. Is this happening to her too? I can't bear to think of her by name. I can't bear the reason I'll fly to Geneva in a few days.

This is why I take my mind back to the natural world. To the deer betting on a new rosebud behind the wrought-iron fence. To the wild turkeys gobbling at a courting male that interrupted their cryptic cackles. To the sneaking coyote obsessed with a limping fawn protected by two determined does. And I get it. For a coyote to keep on living, a limping fawn may die.

Since I arrived in California, a week ago, I remember that I irritated my friend when I complained about my constant coming and going between Vancouver and California—our home for seventeen years and where two of our children live. I also visit my aging parents and relatives in France and take trips with Jim, my husband.

My traveling creates physical and emotional disruptions and moving from France to Switzerland, and back, then to the United States, and finally to Canada, was challenging. But I understand my friend's irritation at my complaining.

In Vancouver, my rather quiet life doesn't compare with her life of hardships. And, here, in California, I enjoy part of the day with three rambunctious grandchildren and a dog in one house, and quiet evenings with my stepdaughter in the other.

As I gaze out the window of the 'quiet house,' the oak trees seem greener and the bark of the redwoods brighter, but it's from the rain that finally fell on the golden hills of the East Bay. The dry grasses will soon morph into a landscape of green pastures and black cattle. The prospect of their return is reassuring, as the evidence that life will go on as usual. Yet *going on* never means that things stay the same.

When the first farmers came to the Far West in the late 1800s, California's rolling hills stayed green through late summer until they imported a Mediterranean type of grass. When the invasion became evident, it was too late; the landscape had morphed into the iconic golden hills we see today. That's what happens with cancer, except that it's an uninvited parasite that doesn't let go, even if only psychologically.

Since then, much else changed too. Large clusters of houses spread on the rolling hills of the vast open space of the San Francisco Bay Area. Yet, here in Danville, the Old Wild West is still present, thanks to the preservation of historic buildings and the shop owners who care enough to keep the spirit going. But it's a new—what I'd call—*work order* out there.

Some people commute to Silicon Valley, abiding by working hours that are never totally on or off, not unlike the California seasons. It's a lifestyle that blurs the boundary between personal and working life and flexibility and availability of time. As if only work and time matter.

I am no stranger to impermanence with my regular trips between Canada, California, France, and Switzerland, where my friend is waiting for me. Nor after mothering a blended family. Nor after graduating from university after a midlife crisis. I tend to resist change now, but by all accounts, whether it's a perennial plant that will die someday or an acquired work culture overcome by a pandemic, much in life is temporary.

My thoughts were cut short by a nap; the afternoon dawdled from seconds into minutes that rushed into hours. Dusk has darkened the garden. In the centuries-old oak tree, the resident owl hoots at the nearing night.

Each day has a beginning and an end, and I am ending this day of February 2014 knowing that, in a few days, I'll be in Geneva to 'accompany' my friend. That's what she said, and I have never done this before. What happens when your friend has a short time to live? I don't know.

I dread that belated rite of passage of a sort. I also stumble on questions with no real answers. Will I be strong enough not to fake hope? We are beyond that. What will our last days together be like? I don't want to think about it. Can anyone tell me?

Most troubling is whether I'll be enough of an 'accompanying' friend on that journey.

Of course, I couldn't have known then that it'd be more of a crusade than a journey. Nor that our differences didn't separate us as much as my friend wanted me to believe. It wouldn't even have made sense that *this* would be her last gift. One that would set me free from the same mold that secretly restrained her. Nor could I have expected that our friendship could help other women understand why they feel the way they do.

Meanwhile, a stubborn case of bronchitis makes me wonder whether this is how health begins to fail sometimes. I struggle with the idea of the impermanence of life because it's bound to the irrevocability of death, and I keep hearing my friend's wise words over the telephone: "Marie-Claude… I can't go against it… It's in my destiny."

CHAPTER 2
Geneva, June 1978

SHE WOULD HAVE called it *serendipitous* that despite living ten minutes away from each other in France we met in Switzerland and became friends for thirty-plus years.

It was my first day in a new job as an executive assistant at Capital International, an investment advisory firm in Geneva. Her name came up while I was on a tour of the offices—she created the statistical graphics displayed on the walls of that department.

Her office was around the corner from mine, so meeting her was only a matter of time.

"*Bonjour!*"

An elegant woman with a confident demeanor stood in front of me, her brown eyes dipping into mine in a friendly way, her smile somewhat forced, guarded even. She stayed at a distance, all the better to give me a full appreciation of her fashion sense.

Whether it was on that day or another, I remember a white blazer, a colorful top, and a set of necklaces akin to the classic Chanel style—black and white pearl strands mingling with gold chains and charms. Her trendy gold earrings were like mine—three semicircles. Her floating black skirt hemmed above the knees revealed shapely legs in shimmering skin-tone nylons. I even took in the buckle—another trend—on her black slingback shoes.

This woman knows her style, I thought.

I didn't anticipate, then, that fashion would become a favorite topic of conversation and our hair somewhat of an obsession.

Her black curls cascaded to her shoulders in a Diane von Furstenberg kind of way, and she even looked like her. As for my then-dark blond bohemian frizzes, I straightened them, inciting her to say soon after we met that I should embrace my natural hair. On that day, I learned to expect her radical opinion on any subject.

As I was also to discover and experience, we both liked to be right, she more adamantly than I—someone had to give in.

"I'm Juliette Volvinsky. My office is around the corner." She held out her hand to invite mine, and we began to chat as people do when they first meet, thinking of something to say. It didn't take her long to size me up.

"Are you nervous about your new job? Is something wrong?" she asked.

Anyone would be a little nervous on the first morning of a new job, but her discerning 'Is something wrong?' took me off guard. I didn't know yet that intuition drove much of Juliette's inquisitive spirit.

"I'm still upset about… uh… about yesterday evening." I hesitated, anticipating that a *yes* or *no* wouldn't satisfy her. "I am not used to city life." I had just moved from a house in the countryside.

"So?" she said, raising her perfectly plucked eyebrows as she noticed my awkwardness.

"Uh, something happened while I was waiting for the elevator." From the tilt of her head, I knew I had to explain. "A man pulled his pants down. Nothing more happened but I was terrified."

"Pfft! These men are not dangerous! So…? What did you do?" Her enthusiasm put me on the spot, and that's how I discovered that Juliette would always demand or give every detail of any situation. It would lead to hilarious, sad, or peculiar stories like this one that broke the ice on that first day.

I had been driving through the security gate of my underground garage when I noticed a man standing there until my rearview mirror showed him heading in my direction. Somewhat troubled—I wasn't used to sharing underground parking with strangers—I parked and then rushed to the elevator lobby. The man showed up shortly after, immediately raising my suspicion. He didn't seem eager to go home at the end of the day. Besides, I felt his stare on me.

I tried to ignore him as I stood by the elevator until he inched so close, I peeked sideways. That's when I saw his belted pants below his hips. Then it all happened fast. Since I failed to push him off-balance as I stepped into the elevator, he quickly blocked the door. I then screamed something like *Go to hell!* Startled, he jolted back and froze, and my shaky finger pressed the button to my floor. As it turned out, this exhibitionist already had a police record.

"You see, I told you! These men are *lavettes*! Don't think about it anymore!" was Juliette's blasé answer. (*Lavette* is French slang for a *weakling*, and a baffling analogy since the literal French translation is *facecloth*.)

I giggled at Juliette's comment and told her I was so shaken I struggled to unlock my apartment's door. After I did, I rushed to the phone to call a friend but dialed the wrong number, three times. Of course, she wanted to know about the anonymous woman I kept calling by mistake.

After apologizing once more to that woman, I was about to hang up when she asked, in a calm and accented voice, why I was so upset. "It can't be *thaat baad*. How *oold* are you?" So, I told her. "*Ooh*, then you must have *seeen thiis* before... *noo*?" Her melodious intonations rose and fell, stretching the keywords to a high note that made me chuckle and would make Juliette laugh herself to tears.

After telling that story, I expected Juliette's blasé attitude in all kinds of circumstances. Life, I learned, had taught her to act that way.

I also quickly understood why Juliette's reaction was so dismissive. I could let go of the incident still on my mind, but she couldn't let go of what was on hers.

"Pfft! Basically... my husband adores me in the morning and hates me in the evening. I can't take it anymore," she said again in that detached way. It was my turn to raise my eyebrows.

"I'm waiting until my youngest daughter turns fifteen. Then I'll divorce him."

This was Juliette's plan when we met more than three decades ago, and she would act upon it in due time. But on that day, I was impressed by her thought-out patience. She 'acknowledged' the thought with a smile and a shrug.

For what would be the first of many lunches together, Juliette suggested a new restaurant, now shut and whose name I forget, on Rue de la Servette, the main artery through Geneva's right bank, close to the office.

At the time, Indian restaurants were still uncommon in Geneva, yet it wasn't my first experience with Indian cuisine—since my student years near London. But it was for Juliette, who still declared she liked spicy food and ordered *devil* butter chicken. I went for *mild*.

Of course, her eyes widened at the first bite, her mouth opening as if something alive had to come out of it. But determined to stand by her word, Juliette endured the rest of her meal thanks to heaping spoons of chutney and numerous cups of tea loaded with sugar.

Juliette could be defiant.

Despite this inauspicious introduction, Indian food would become a part of her life, and a story I'd share.

Thirty-six years of friendship, a third of some people's lives, went by quickly. So much happened that it often seems like it's someone else's story. In a way, it is because the past is gone. And what's left of anyone's life will keep unfolding until it's meant to stop, on its *own* terms.

CHAPTER 3

Getting to Know Juliette

JULIETTE'S STORY OF course began long before we met. She never talked much about the younger Juliette but now and then revealed parts of her earlier life.

She was born and raised in Paris until she left for California in the sixties. She was always evasive as to why she interrupted her brief studies at the Université de la Sorbonne. I assumed she fancied another type of life.

There, she landed a job in Monterey—at the Defense Language Institute. There, it also didn't take long until she fell head over heels for Dimitri, a charismatic Russian raised in China. The handsome man spoke seven languages and was fifteen years her senior. After emigrating to California, he married an opera singer, had a son, and divorced later.

Juliette and Dimitri happened to lay eyes on each other on her first day at the institute. They were arguing about a parking space, and he was furious that this young and sassy newcomer with a quirky accent had the audacity to park in his space. Worse than that, she thought it was no big deal. But Dimitri soon faced a bigger deal when Juliette walked into the classroom. She was the new French teacher.

They married, had three children, moved to Paris, and then

to Switzerland where Dimitri worked as an interpreter at the United Nations. Their strong personalities, different cultures, Dimitri's convoluted background, and his penchant for alcohol—and Juliette's inner conflicts as I was to find out later—led to troubles. Dishes were smashed, and damaged doors remained the evidence of their explosive marriage decades later.

Dimitri's profession also made matters worse.

Interpreters work in simultaneous oral communication and have only a split second to convert an idea into their own words. Confined in booths to help their concentration, it's a stressful job: a misunderstanding can have a serious impact on international relations. When Dimitri and his colleagues were on recess, standby, or meetings were deferred, the bar was the interpreters' informal lounge. Alcohol was part of the working arsenal in the sixties and a bad combination for Juliette and Dimitri's relationship, and the worst for their family life.

After Juliette and I became friends in the late seventies, we socialized with our husbands on a few occasions. Dimitri and Jim didn't see eye to eye but obliged. Dimitri was often confrontational and judgmental, and Jim held his own.

One revealing memory of Dimitri and Juliette's married life is of a weekend in Megève, a quaint Alpine ski resort in Haute-Savoie, and a one-hour drive from Geneva where we lived at the time. We had invited them and another couple—Marianne and Jean-Paul—to the chalet we rented. Jim and I went downhill skiing, and the two couples had their first experience with cross-country skiing. The end of the day brought us by the fireplace, chatting and enjoying a few drinks before dinner.

Jean-Paul talked about the upcoming publication of his book, *The ABCs of Jazz*—a biographical index of American jazz singers. Passionate about jazz and blues music, in the sixties, he organized European tours for African-American artists. This piqued Dimitri's curiosity, as did the fact that Jean-Paul had an impressive collection of LPs and singles.

Dimitri was a worldly, artistically inclined man and a self-taught painter and sculptor. He was charming until the conversations veered to our day in the snow, and he became agitated, alcohol turning him into an aggressive character, who recalled being left behind among the trees.

"It was my first time on any kind of skis… Can you understand that? It was, well… unimaginably difficult. I could barely catch my breath, I felt like… I was choking! That's why I had trouble following you… and you… and you." He hurled each "you" while pointing a finger at Marianne, then Jean-Paul, and then holding it up at Juliette.

That unforgettable scene was like a rendition of a comedic act at first, or somewhat akin to a conductor guiding the orchestra. But what seemed like a joke quickly turned into brash blaming, although nothing was said—yet—to trigger his loss of control. We were all perplexed, except for Juliette, who looked embarrassed. Her husband's ranting could turn ugly but in trying to dissipate the tension she added fuel to the fire instead.

"Oh… wait a minute! It was difficult for all of us! What did you expect? You don't exercise and you smoke! It wasn't a competition… it was *so-oo* beautiful out there." Juliette's attempt at trivializing Dimitri's outburst was in sheer contrast with her contrite smile. She had to know that her blunt criticism would blow his fuse, but it was as if she was inexplicably conditioned to act that way.

Dimitri's face turned red. A strand of salt-and-pepper hair

sliced his face as he stood up, verbally lashing out at Juliette, and I forgot what else he said. Anger does what anger does, and as I would hear from her on several occasions, at home he may have turned violent.

Seconds stood unnervingly empty until Jean-Paul volunteered to downplay the incident. Calmly, and never at a loss for witty improvisation, he recalled "struggling like *hell* in that otherwise *heavenly* winter scenery," emphasizing these words while smoking the same pipe that had made *him* puff equally hard out there. Dimitri froze and then sat down, a sneering grin on his face.

I would often see the same anxious expression on Juliette's face until she left him a few years later. After her youngest daughter turned fifteen.

Juliette was attracted to a dashing and enigmatic man and Dimitri to a beautiful and spirited woman. Their effervescent personalities demanded many compromises, but Dimitri's drinking demanded more than that. She left him for the sake of her family's safety.

Despite the hardships in her life, Juliette shielded herself from painful thoughts, never projecting herself as a victim. It worked until her unconscious mind caught up with her; aging deepened her loneliness and cancer weakened her resolve.

Then years of holding back would drag out a secret I didn't know she had.

CHAPTER 4

In Those Days

AFTER WE MOVED to the United States in the mid-eighties, I only saw Juliette during my visits to my family in France unless she visited us.

Sometimes, we had lunch or dinner in a quaint village where I enjoyed the seasonal food I was craving. Simple dishes made from local ingredients: plump white asparagus in springtime, scrumptious fruit tarts in the summertime, buttery chestnuts in the fall, and juicy cardoons—the stems of a plant related to the artichoke—in wintertime, to name a few of my favorite foods.

As for the legendary frog legs, *fresh* might now mean *trucked alive from Turkey* whereas the cheaper ones are imported frozen from Indonesia. I only have them in Bresse, near Lyon, the cradle of both French gastronomy and my maternal family.

Other than going to a restaurant, Juliette and I might have gone shopping, but we never went to a show—we couldn't have talked. As for walking in the countryside, it was never on her mind. Besides, I never saw Juliette wear shoes even close to sneakers.

High heels were her favorites, even on boots. One year, we bought the same pair of red leather boots, in a Western style. After our move to California and I went back to school, these red boots got the attention of the psychology professor; she commented that only a woman who owns more than one pair would buy red boots. I was reminded of that story after seeing Juliette wear hers on my next visit to France. "Had she lived in Switzerland where we wear boots almost half the year, she might have owned more than one pair too," Juliette said with her usual wit. After retirement, Juliette surrendered to wearing comfortable shoes although with a twist: color, print, shape, whatever made them stand out.

Our time together always went by too quickly. We shared our thoughts and feelings as women freely do. We had animated conversations about politics and pop culture. Sometimes, Juliette vented about her cantankerous mother, and I shared my frustration at my elderly parents' implied expectations during my visits; plus, those I created or placed on my myself. She also told me about her latest argument with Corinne, her daughter.

I often listened more than I talked because Juliette lived alone and was always eager to speak. She didn't email regularly in between my visits; unlike me, Juliette wasn't an eager writer, but she was an editor.

In those days, after I rang the bell Juliette opened her front door, welcoming me with her signature half-smile.

Her approach seemed conceited to someone who didn't know her. The Parisian in her stood composed, her clothes and makeup were perfect for the time of day, and she'd stand there as if *she* were making an entrance. I always praised her for being *en beauté*—looking beautiful—and the first thing she commented back on was her hair.

At times, if she noticed the slightest hesitation in the way I looked at it, she might admit that something was a little off: her hair was shorter or straighter or curlier than usual. If the blunder was evident, an endless explanation followed, somewhat like the six questions of journalism: *who* the stylist was; *what*, *why*, and *when* it happened; *where* the salon was; and *how* it could have been prevented. In her view, the stylist didn't follow her, reportedly and pun aside, 'clear-cut' explanations. The story ended with the fact that she'd never visit that hair salon again.

Juliette usually let me precede her into her stylish yet cozy living room, expecting me to immediately notice anything new. If I didn't, she waited until I did. And if I still had no clue, she couldn't understand why. Never mind that some six months had gone by since my last trip to France.

Her home interior began as white as a blank canvas; the walls, tiled floor, and furniture, all were white. Then two large Oriental rugs and collectibles gave the tone of her décor like the accents on French words. It was a muted palette of autumn landscapes, dimming sunsets, and sun-kissed grasses on sandy dunes, enhanced with bright splashes here and there. It was at once monochromatic but not. It could catch one off-guard, like Juliette's personality.

She concocted the placement of her furniture and displayed objects from the best angle. And she had a story about each one.

She would explain in a nonchalant yet captivating delivery why a new painting looked better *here* rather than *there*. Some were by artists she'd met at a private gathering or an art gallery. Others were bought on the cheap from street vendors in exotic places. Regardless of value, choosing the frame involved days of indecision.

To someone else, she may have appeared obsessive in her attention to shape, subject, and colors, but it was her way to be in the moment, to connect closely with her space, to push back the somber thoughts. In that sense, she was a misunderstood woman. A woman who hid her broken heart.

CHAPTER 5
The Photograph

AT THIS VERY moment, and in between two coughing spells, I am still nestling on the sofa, hugging a knitted throw, nuzzling its loops to pacify my heavy heart.

Last August, six months ago, Juliette's appearance in a photograph posted on Facebook troubled me. At the time, I hadn't seen her since my last trip to France, in the spring.

She had recently returned from a trip to New York with her three granddaughters: the French one and the American twins. The twins' mother was her youngest daughter, who lived in the United States and who, as I'll explain later, died tragically some ten years earlier. Juliette did what her late daughter couldn't do anymore, keep her French and American families connected.

The photograph posted by one of the girls showed them sitting on a bench and something was wrong.

Juliette looked unkempt, thinner, and weary. Her face had shadows I'd never noticed before. And most shocking was her limp-looking hair. I never saw her like this in a photograph and seldom in real life. There was also something unfamiliar in the way she was hunched over. Not wanting to infer that she was exhausted from keeping up with three teenagers, I concluded that photographs can be misleading, but I noticed a difference.

I called Juliette from Vancouver after she returned home, shortly after seeing the photograph. The trip was difficult. She never felt well, even before she left—uncomfortable, bloated.

At the time, it would never have dawned on me to associate her apparent weight loss with one of the symptoms of pancreatic cancer, and although I knew that yellowish skin and eyes are signs of jaundice, therefore illness, it wasn't visible on a simple snapshot. I never suspected that what followed would happen to Juliette.

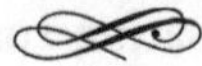

LIKE MOST PEOPLE in such circumstances, I learned online the basic facts about pancreatic cancer. According to the Cleveland Clinic, jaundice is caused by a high level of bilirubin, a yellow-orange pigment in the bile, the concentration of which can cause a tumor, cancerous or not. And from Johns Hopkins Medicine, that jaundice is only painful in pancreatic cancer, the tumor in the head of the pancreas blocking the bile duct.

Tragically, and of course unbeknownst to Juliette at the time, and as happens in approximately eighty percent of pancreatic cancer cases, hers had already metastasized. Every case is unique, and statistics can be confusing, but "By the time you bring this to a physician, it's too late," Dr. Anirban Maitra stated, in the 2012 article, "Jack Andraka, the Teen Prodigy of Pancreatic Cancer," on the *Smithsonian* magazine website. The point is, there is no standard test for early diagnosis.

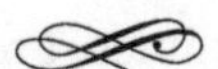

BEFORE HER NEW York trip, Juliette felt uncomfortable enough to call her family physician; the prospect of being sick was a normal concern. He gave her one piece of advice, over the telephone, *take a mild laxative*. But since her return from New York, eating was painful and she was losing weight, except on her belly.

When I finally associated her look in the photograph with the troubling symptoms she described, I immediately remembered a Vancouver friend—similar symptoms turned for the worse.

On that day, our conversation ended with her promise to see a doctor, any doctor since hers was now on summer vacation. But nothing was new the next day; Juliette had decided to wait for her physician's return. I sensed her worry and hung up the telephone with the premonition that our conversations might never be the same again. Life as we knew it had changed.

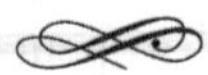

DURING THAT LONG-GONE weekend in the mountains with our friends, it wouldn't have occurred to me to think of what the future held for all of us. It's natural not to think of death when we are young, yet young people die every day.

Fate would take Dimitri first, years after he retired in Slovenia, married his Croatian girlfriend, and had a daughter. Then Jean-Paul was to pass during heart surgery, in 2005. And now, Juliette is in the abyss of cancer.

It has been six months since we first talked about her symptoms. And since that last summer, I feel as if we are even farther apart than before.

I am here, on my stepdaughter's sofa near San Francisco, watching a squirrel scuttle headfirst down the trunk of a redwood tree as if it were going the wrong way. Yet this is what squirrels do. And Juliette is there, lying in a hospital bed in Geneva. I try to imagine how she feels. I find I can't. I have bronchitis; she has cancer. Unlike the squirrel, *she* is going the wrong way.

I also feel guilty about only needing some rest to get better, in the comfort of a nice home, while gazing at nature. But my gaze is not empty.

The day that Juliette called her doctor had come, and I'd heard nothing more from her. I'd tried to reach her for three days with phone calls, messages, and emails. Even her neighbor friend appeared to be absent. I hadn't seen Juliette's daughter for years and although I'd seen her son a few years back, I had no contact information.

During that weekend, it finally occurred to me to do a Facebook search for Juliette's daughter, Corinne, but her account showed little activity. I followed up with a search for Corinne's daughter who then alerted her mother of my attempts at getting in touch.

Tuesday, August 14, 2013

Dear Marie-Claude,

I have tried to call you but got your voicemail [she had called my American flip phone]. *You will find a confusing message. I am glad we can communicate, so I can answer your questions. Juliette was in such pain from the bloating she was indeed admitted to the hospital last Friday. She had an emergency procedure to remove over three liters* [approximately one gallon] *of fluid from her abdomen. This type of fluid is usually a sign of an advanced stage of cancer. An ultrasound revealed a tumor on one ovary. The tumor was removed yesterday during a two-hour surgical procedure, as well as metastatic lesions in her intestine.*

My mother is now recovering from this painful surgery. She will need chemotherapy and probably further surgeries. We are waiting for the result of the biopsy. Despite everything, she faces the situation with courage and even some humor. You can contact her directly at [the hospital number]. *Hugs and best regards to the family.*

Corinne

I called the hospital the next day and found Juliette surprisingly talkative. She was relieved that the surgery was over and recovering before the 'next one.' She sounded as if all would be well afterward, but I didn't like to hear what I already knew from Corinne's message.

It made no sense to me that she would need another surgery. Why had everything suspect not been removed? The evidence of something worse was looming.

I was also baffled that Juliette, who was always curious about the whys and why-nots of any situation, didn't ask more questions of the surgeon, nor made any such comment to me. Instead, she gave me a detailed account of what happened.

Juliette had called her doctor on that fateful Friday, and again a few days later, complaining that the laxatives provided no relief, her abdomen was still swollen, and her discomfort was increasing. This time, he prescribed *patience*.

"You won't believe what else he said." The sarcastic tone of her voice prepared me not to believe what he had said: *she ate too many hamburgers during her trip to the United States.* Recalling his arrogant joke revived Juliette's anger. She was furious about his mockery of her discomfort and demanded a consultation.

She knew something was terribly wrong when the doctor's face froze as he examined her. He then gave her a sealed envelope and ordered that she immediately go to the ER, admitting that he was wrong all along. "*Bien sûr!* (Of course!) If anyone knows what's wrong with *my* body, it's *me*, not *you*," was her reaction. This was one of her unforgettable railleries through her cancer ordeal.

She had then driven herself to Hôpital de la Tour in Meyrin, a Geneva suburb located fifteen minutes from her doctor's office. Terrified, she waited for her turn in the waiting room, glancing at the envelope that sealed her fate. The receptionist opened it and looked at Juliette in a learned inscrutable way that didn't fool Juliette; the woman knew more than she did. Juliette forgot what happened next. While she talked, I envisioned her trip to the hospital, alone and worried about the gravity of her condition.

When I called Juliette again two days later, her words took my breath away—cancer… chemotherapy. My heart sank. My friend did have cancer.

The sequence of what followed became a blur. Further surgery didn't happen, but chemotherapy started, and with it the side effects from poisoning the whole body to destroy the malicious cells.

Staying in touch was complicated due to the nine-hour time difference between France and North America's Pacific Coast. Then, when I called her home, she was in the hospital. And when I called the hospital one day, she was in a convalescent care clinic. She went to the hospital every two weeks for chemotherapy, but as she was too sick and dehydrated to stay home, her children had her readmitted to the hospital.

When we did talk, we tried to ignore what lay ahead, chatting about other things rather than her illness. It gave us the illusion that nothing had changed. We discussed the news in our tumultuous world. We even touched on fashion, which reminded me of past conversations.

Fashion was over the top and unflattering even for fit, grown-up women like us. We wanted to be stylish, not a caricature of our younger selves. After I moved to the United States, in the mid-eighties, Juliette even commented on my "American style," claiming I had "lost my French flair and was dressing *so-oo* conservatively."

And Juliette still talked about her hair. "It was getting so long, I trimmed it myself. I now have side bangs and it looks *so-oo* much better." As if better hair suddenly revived her hope of recovery. "For sure, a stylist would have cut it too short," she added. Ah, she had a point—I have much to say about this myself.

That day, she sounded pleased to "look healthier, if not on the inside at least on the outside." If one thing could lift her mood, it would be a good hair day.

CHAPTER 6
A Happier-Ending Crisis

I WAS BACK home in Vancouver after my trip to California when September of 2013 brought some new perspectives with Corinne's phone call and then her email.

She was exhausted. And as if her mother's condition wasn't enough, she had a cancerous skin lesion removed from her back… And she had the same oncologist as her mother… And she wanted to divorce… And she worried about her children… It was a lot to take in over the telephone, but I was attentive to her need for a supportive ear.

Corinne didn't talk much about her mother that day, but she did about her marriage. She was the frustrated breadwinner for her family of four, and weary of her husband's lack of support, something that equally frustrated her mother. Juliette's exasperation over the inequality in her daughter's marriage wasn't news to me. From what I understood, her son-in-law was a kind but laid-back artist who wouldn't envision any supplemental work.

I tried to help Corinne put things in perspective. Under the circumstances, no one would benefit from her drastic decision to get a divorce, not even her.

I followed up by messaging Corinne the next day. I didn't want Juliette to know about our phone conversation. As perceptive as she was, giving a casual reason for Corinne calling me would make no sense to her and my evasive answer would only lead to her suspicion.

I also acknowledged Corinne's frustration, reminding her that instead of focusing on separating from her husband she needed to focus: first on her mother while she was still alive, then on taking care of herself so she could stay strong, then on paying attention to her teenage children, and lastly on her marriage. She admitted her tendency to control; perhaps she could let go a little. I wasn't in her situation, but these priorities seemed reasonable.

The next day, I messaged Corinne again. We were back in Vancouver, but my husband was hospitalized. After a weekend at a spa to celebrate my birthday, nasty bacteria lodged under the skin of his leg and generated a serious infection. Corinne replied a few days later.

September 14, 2013

Dear Marie-Claude,

Thank you for having been a good listener on the phone the other day. […] I am thinking about you as much as I know your thoughts are with us. […] Thank you for keeping our last conversation to yourself. Since then, things have been much better. I can't believe all I have shared with you whereas we don't know each other well. I felt your closeness. I am afraid that exhaustion and anxiety made me dramatic that day, not to forget my Slavic genes.

My husband had to react and take much upon himself after the doctor prescribed some time off work because of my exhaustion. It has helped me calm down and put things in perspective. [...] Disagreements are inevitable in a marriage, but we have known each other for so long; in the end, they remind us that no relationship is perfect. If there is still love, it will be fine. I can't imagine us living apart. I must, however, let go of some of my obsolete expectations; it's not easy to change.

In a strange way, this is what I see happening with Juliette. She is in a paradoxical state of positive metamorphosis: her horizon has shrunk but her compassion for others has grown. She is still shocked by what is happening to her, but she is happy to see how close we all have become. [...] My daughter told me that she is sad, yet at the same time, she is now aware that things happen in life and that all we can do is give love. [...] The family is more united than we have ever been. At the same time, it's hard to accept that we have found this space of tenderness because of cancer. I am losing a mother, and I am finding one, more than I have ever felt before. To this, I would add that listening to you talking about her has helped me see her differently.

Yesterday, I had an appointment with my oncologist. [...] He will still do an ultrasound to be sure. Then I told him that my mother was his patient, too. He shook his head and said that what was happening was dramatic. I am telling you this, unbeknownst to Mom. The real problem is a rare carcinoma; her body produces a type of mucus that makes chemotherapy ineffective. [...] She is very alert and careful about the medicine that is given to her since she is severely allergic to some chemicals. She won't take anything that is not in its packaging, to be sure that no mistake is

made. She is courageous and upbeat but with a sweetness that I didn't know she had. As for me, all my anger and resentment toward her have been replaced by love, and hope. Nothing will ever take this away and I know that she feels the same way. It's both sad and beautiful. We will visit her tomorrow, and I will give her a hug for you. [...] This is a long message. [...]. Meanwhile, I wish you courage and patience as Jim gets good care until he can go home. [...]
Hugs,
Corinne

Her poignant message brought me to tears. There was so much to think about. She saw the positive side of her marriage just as she was about to leave it. Juliette wouldn't get better, but the family had rallied around her.

I was especially moved by "a sweetness I didn't know she had" and "her anger and resentment were replaced by love and hope." Mother and daughter were mending years of a confrontational relationship.

Two weeks later, Juliette was back at home and enjoying moments of regained energy. She could eat and take short walks in her garden. In typical Juliette fashion, she even reorganized some of her home décor. She hoped to drive again soon. In three weeks, she would know whether the chemotherapy had worked. She remained "mentally strong, open, and natural."

This news brought back the Juliette I knew. I even imagined her in her bathrobe, plucking a faded bloom in her garden. As for my husband, he too was mending and could drive himself to his daily clinic appointments. Life was almost back to normal.

September of 2013 had been a roller coaster of emotions that deeply connected an unlikely threesome: Juliette, her daughter, and me. I hadn't seen Corinne in years, yet we were bonding in surprising ways.

From her home-front problems, Corinne also realized that the trees look greener when we imagine seeing them for the last time.

CHAPTER 7

France, September 2013

JULIETTE EXPECTED SURGERIES and chemotherapy to restore her health. But as she quickly learned, cancer had already invaded her liver. "I hope you're not going to tell me that I only have six months to live." Her oncologist's reply was evasive, but the cancellation of the second surgery was his unspoken estimation. Her new reality was the countdown to the end of her life.

When I visited my parents in France, in mid-October 2013, Juliette was on a gruelling regimen of chemotherapy. After each treatment, she rested at home, trying to prepare mentally and physically for the next round.

The morning after my late arrival, and after getting no response at her home, I called the hospital. She had been readmitted for dehydration the day before. She hadn't seen her daughter for a few days; Corinne had conjunctivitis, and her whole family was sick. I rushed to the hospital eager to be with my friend.

When I walked into her room, she was throwing up in a bowl. She looked pale and thin. After I could embrace her, her familiar brown eyes went right through mine, but I held her stare. I knew she expected the truth. Yes, she had lost weight. Yes, she looked sick. Yes, her hair wasn't at its best. And yes, this whole thing was the pits. But what mattered now was to fight, one day at a time.

"It won't be easy... cancer moved to my pancreas."

I heard her, but don't remember whether I said anything. We both knew the poor odds of recovering from pancreatic cancer. I knew of the metastases from Corinne's message so it shouldn't have been a complete shock, but my 'face-to-face' with her spoken words was paralyzing.

Before Juliette's diagnosis, I sometimes brought up with her the subject of medical checkups. She was either evasive, dismissive, or defensive; she used to say she was in good health and seldom sick. Yet, her defiance didn't entirely work against her.

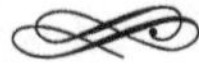

UNBEKNOWNST TO ME at first, I learned from the PanCAN's website that "the pancreas is located deep in the abdomen, so doctors usually cannot see or feel the tumor during a physical exam." Furthermore: "Pancreatic cancer symptoms are not always obvious and usually develop over time."

That Juliette's cancer spread so fast wasn't unusual: "[...] pancreatic cancer can progress very quickly from stage I (localized within the pancreas) to stage IV (metastatic disease) in an average of 1.3 years."

Of course, Juliette wanted as much remission time as possible, but unlike people who experience a better outcome, even years-long survival, her specific stage IV, at the time of diagnosis, and her age, would give her only seven months to live.

There are two reasons for this: Not only are 'warning signs rare' but "there's no standard early detection test for the general population." The point is: "It is critical to develop early detection tools."

CT scans detect pancreatic cysts, the incidence of which is on the rise, occurring in 'twenty-five percent of people over the age of seventy.' The good news is that not all cysts are cancerous and 'surgically removing high-risk ones significantly enhances a patient's survival.'

Pancreatic cancer is a complex illness.

No matter the facts, it dawned on me that unless an incurable illness strikes someone we love, we don't relate to the urgency of finding a cure.

As for other risk factors, Juliette was always slim, so obesity wasn't one. That she looked thinner in the past years might be a result of aging, some women losing body mass, and some gaining weight. She once was a heavy smoker but quit in her forties, and she was never exposed to dangerous chemicals in her line of work—another risk factor.

A FEW DAYS later, I observed the clear liquid of chemotherapy drip from the bag into the intravenous device connected to Juliette's arm, and from there to her bloodstream where it would get into a fierce fight with the cancerous cells, destroying the healthy ones too.

Minutes later, she began to shiver. The nurse brought one more blanket and another, to no avail. A cold wave overcame her each time, Juliette said. At the time, I didn't know that *cold dysesthesia* is a side effect of chemotherapy medication.

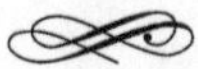

As I revise this manuscript, some comparisons give more perspective.

Five years *before* Juliette's diagnosis, actor Patrick Swayze was diagnosed with stage IV pancreatic cancer. In *Worth Fighting For*, his wife Lisa Niemi Swayze recalls the sip of Champagne on New Year's Eve 2008 that caused unusual stomach pain. She had noticed that he had 'been hitting the Tums pretty regularly,' but didn't worry—he had a sensitive digestive system. But he also hadn't been feeling well, losing twenty pounds until he noticed his yellowish eyes. He fought the illness with experimental therapies and, despite the recurring infections that floored him, met his acting commitments. "He died on September 14, 2009, after a twenty-one-month battle," Niemi Swayze writes.

I don't know whether Juliette ever resorted to antacid tablets, a need that shouldn't be ignored even if most users are never diagnosed with pancreatic cancer.

Unlike Patrick Swayze, Juliette gave up treatment, unable to sustain the physical ordeal of additional therapies.

Six years *after* Juliette's diagnosis, in March 2019, television personality Alex Trebek was also diagnosed with pancreatic cancer. In an essay published by the magazine *Health*, his wife Jean recalls noticing that "his skin color was off," followed by his admission to stomach pains, and a CT scan revealing stage IV pancreatic cancer. Experimental therapies let him survive for twenty months, to the admiration of his *Jeopardy!* fans, his television game show.

Sadly, from 2008 to 2019, the symptoms were still silent for early intervention.

On the positive side, PanCAN points out that over the past decade, the five-year survival rate for pancreatic cancer patients increased from six to twelve percent—it was six percent in 2014 when Juliette died and is twelve percent in 2023. It is expected to be thirteen percent by 2024.

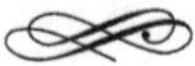

THE RAPID OUTCOME of my friend's incurable illness shocked me into understanding the fragility of life, in a collective way. Sometimes, we must fight for it for ourselves and sometimes for others too.

CHAPTER 8

Understanding Juliette

After her divorce, Juliette rented a flat, then bought an apartment, and then a duplex in a small housing development in one of the rural communities of Pays de Gex—in this case, the word *pays* means *land*, not *country*, and is the terminology for a territorial subdivision such as a former sovereign barony, for example.

Her charming duplex in peaceful surroundings, stood along a single, no-exit lane, with a backyard facing a pasture and nonchalant cows.

"I must admit, they are the perfect neighbors," Juliette once said as we relaxed in the shade of the extended eaves of the roof. "You know, their destiny is to graze and graze, and graze again so we get milk, and when they are too old, they go for a ride and may well end up in spaghetti Bolognese." Her voice stuttered into a laugh as we stared back at the cows' entitled gazes and silent ruminating. Out of derision, Juliette could say the darnedest things sometimes and pondered destiny in unexpected ways.

Juliette's garden was another topic of conversation, and one we have in common.

A typical home gardener, Juliette enjoyed giving a tour of her blooms and bushes.

In the front garden, she'd point to the white rose 'French lace' in a circular flower bed. It was a gift from me, so come May or June she shared on the telephone when it was in full bloom. Next was her collection of potted annuals for shade, on the side of the house with no afternoon sun.

She'd explain why she chose one plant over another and disagree over deciduous versus non-deciduous bushes with the gardener-for-hire, often changing her mind as he dug a hole, transplanted, or trimmed.

There was no cutting the garden tour short; it had to end in the backyard where lush bushes occupied the sides so her narrow lawn would visually extend to the pasture. And of course, her patch of red roses got her full attention.

We agreed that having a garden is like having a friend. When the garden needs you, you better respond, or wilted plants will be the retaliation. In exchange, the garden always soothes the blues in your heart.

Our gardening fashion sense, however, was quite different. It's almost a matter of *Tell me what you wear in the garden, and I'll tell you who you are*. The proverbial *Tell me who your friends are, and I'll tell you who are,* could apply here too.

I like getting dirty in the garden, it cleanses my mind and connects me with Mother Nature. All fashion sense is gone from the large-brimmed hat that replaced various baseball caps, to my black socks inside grimy white Crocs—my red Western-style rubber boots are now a keepsake.

I wasn't like Judy, my former Vancouver neighbor-friend and fashionista gardener, who made me feel a tad self-conscious. She carried herself with style as if she were still a commercial actor now modeling garden accessories—a real garden tool bag, proper clogs, and the color of her visor matching her clothing. Not so for Juliette and me, not in the garden.

Juliette's unique style was often to deadhead or weed early in the morning, in her bathrobe, her cup of coffee cooling on the outdoor table. I know this because when I'd call from my parents' house, this is what she was often doing in summertime. I never asked, but should someone ring her doorbell, I bet she'd crawl under a bush from fear of being found. Most women understand that.

When Juliette talked about gardening, it was from personal expertise. The only way to care for roses and winterize geraniums was her way: You prune the roses in January and throw away what's left of the soggy geraniums after the first frost got them.

She was proud of her roses and furious that the neighbor's cat liked them too. Despite various deterrents, the cat's potty spot was Juliette's patch of cheerful red roses. "French cats like a luxury," she'd say.

One year, I gave her a repellent called Not Tonight Deer, which I used on my roses in California. The putrescent smell should repulse a French cat attracted by the delicate fragrance of roses, but after a sniff and her disgusted look at me, I confessed. It worked for the deer, but I couldn't stand the smell either.

Juliette connected with her outdoor space often with obsession. Her attention to detail was on alert even when we chatted in her backyard. The conversation would stop, and she'd leap from her chair to straighten an object on the garden shelves against the house wall or to snip a spent bloom that had previously escaped her scrutiny. It never bothered me; I am familiar with that urge. Jim often suggested it could wait, really. I am guilty of giving in to that urge with anyone's geraniums, although Juliette only had to summon me once to leave hers alone.

Ah, there is a carnal satisfaction in the snapping sound of a strong geranium stem, but it must be done at its base, or that pleasing pop won't happen.

Transplanting old bushes or planting new ones was always a lengthy exercise in critical thinking for Juliette. She often turned into stories her visits to the Jardiland garden center, where her grandchildren enjoyed looking at the fish and rabbits for sale.

Juliette's garden satisfied her creativity and soothed her loneliness. Weeding or planting is an instant gratification. There is no expectation of someone else's willingness; she alone held the physical and emotional reins of her sanctuary.

During that visit in October 2013—one month after her surgery and five months before she'd die—Juliette looked dazed at times. She was trying to come to terms with the unexpected turn her life had taken.

There was also a shift in her preferences, like buying the best of eiderdowns whereas she always insisted that blankets were better than those expensive down comforters.

Juliette could be thrifty at times, then splurge on something that struck her fancy, of course after much deliberation. As she commented on the cuddliness of the comforter, I complimented her on her choice. I was grateful for the pleasure that softened her face and sad that it'd be the last time she bought something by choice.

Another significant change was Juliette not caring about clothes anymore, resorting to pull-string pants instead—anything else was either too big or felt too tight on her bloated belly. The rest of her body mass melted away from a lack of nutrition due to her pancreas's inability to help digestion, regulate blood sugar, and convert food into fuel for the cells.

Fashion had been a passion and discussing it was now something of the past.

Then one day out of the blue, Juliette blurted out what her ninety-nine-year-old mother said after she informed her of her sickness: she was "old enough to be sick." These were scathing words, even in the context of their ongoing conflicts.

Speechless at first from the way our conversion veered that day, I commented that her elderly mother was either suffering from dementia or hadn't grappled with the gravity of her illness.

"I told her I have *cancer*." Her pained scream of disgust for that word was so shocking, I wondered what caused such hatred between mother and daughter.

Juliette often raged about her mother, who she said always found new ways to hurt her but always praised her brother—Juliette's only sibling. But on that day, Juliette hoped for a little compassion, even from a mother who, from what I know, was never affectionate.

I never met Juliette's mother, whom she visited once or twice a year in Paris, out of a daughter's duty to her elderly mother, nothing more, as she implied. Her mother's nastiness was another source of grief in Juliette's life. Sadly, Juliette's toxic bond with her mother spilled over to her relationship with her daughter, like water over the color pigments on the painter's paper. Although Juliette and Corinne got closer since Juliette's diagnosis, Juliette and her mother never would.

Could she ever share with anyone else her hatred of her mother as viscerally as she did with me? I should have known that there was more to it than she was willing to tell.

To Juliette's relief, and as I will share later, her mother died shortly before she did. As for her father, all I knew, then, was that he was deceased.

There were so many convolutions in Juliette's life that I had to accept my difficulty in understanding her completely.

CHAPTER 9
A Complicated Day

OCTOBER TURNED TOO quickly into November; it was time for me to leave France and return home to Vancouver. Juliette was feeling better, so we spent my last day there doing errands. The prospect of some accomplishments energized her, and our time together boosted her morale just in time before the ordeal of her next treatment. At this point, Juliette still had some hope but whether it was for a long-term survival or short remission, we never discussed it.

First on our to-do list was Juliette's internet provider in Ferney-Voltaire, the city indeed named after the eighteenth-century philosopher and whose former country castle is open to visitors. She had to cancel her contract since she no longer needed that service. It struck me that this was another step that cut her off from the life she knew.

Next was a twenty-minute drive to Manor Shopping Center in Chavannes-de-Bogis. It's in Switzerland, but only a few minutes away from the French border, at Divonne-Les-Bains, a quaint spa resort with a lake, casino, horserace track, and pricey real estate.

On that sunny autumnal day, Juliette's commanding way made me take a shortcut through quaint French and Swiss villages instead of staying on the main road. The speed limit on the narrow streets gave her plenty of time to enjoy the seasonal sights. The bright pumpkins lingering in otherwise fading gardens, the dry leaves fluffing the roadside, and on the mountainside, the flamboyant deciduous foliage contrasting with the dark evergreens. I didn't mind the other so-called *shortcut* leading onto a dirt road with muddy clumps and dead ending at a freshly plowed plot.

Our lighter-hearted mood, however, disappeared when we walked into the shopping mall.

Juliette walked slowly, attentive to each store as if she wanted to encapsulate everything she saw. From time to time, she made a heartbreaking, thought-provoking comment that troubled me despite my confident composure.

When we walked by a *boutique*—a small, independent clothing store—she said she bought nice outfits there. I weighed the past tense of her comment and guessed what was on her mind from the tone of her voice—it would never happen again.

I once more tried to imagine how I'd feel if I knew I was looking at things for the last time. I was sad and incredulous that this was true for my friend.

At a loss to soften the moment, I mentioned one of her jackets. Whether she bought it there, I didn't recall, but it'd give her something else to think about. I should have known better.

"I did *not* buy it here," she snapped, emphasizing *not* as if she knew I was trying to make conversation. I vaguely heard her say where she bought it and for what occasion but, disconcerted by the tone of her voice, I wasn't attentive to the details. "It would have been too expensive here unless it was on sale." She did make her point.

It was almost noon, so I suggested we have lunch, also a reason for her to rest.

I ordered what she did, then watched her take occasional bites of a quiche Lorraine and sparingly select the leaves of a mixed greens salad. I didn't have the heart to indulge in one of my favorite autumnal desserts in Switzerland, called *Mont Blanc*.

It's a sweetened chestnut *purée* turned into *vermicelles* (like the *vermicelli* pasta—meaning worms!) and crowned with nothing less than heavy cream flavored with Kirsch brandy. When chestnuts are not in season, in the spring, my favorite dessert is a crisp meringue from Gruyères with a heap of double cream and loads of *fraises des bois*—Alpine strawberries. And if the berries are not in season either, any very buttery pastry will do.

Passing on that dessert wasn't important—I could still have it some other time, only not this time. But *other times* would always remind me of that day. When I was losing my friend.

We then crossed the border back to France where our last errand was at the megastore Carrefour. That's where and when my phone rang.

My mother was at the hospital with my eighty-six-year-old dad. He'd fallen into the small fountain basin while trying to save a frog. It wasn't a joke.

I had tried to dissuade my dad from cleaning that basin again: the goldfish might prefer to hibernate in less than crystal-clear waters. I wasn't sure about that, only wanting him to take it easy, but you don't tell my dad he shouldn't do something that "has worked well for half a century," as he would say.

And so, after my dad scooped the fish out of the water and dropped it into a bucket, the resident frog jumped from a bush and into the basin that my dad just drained. Fearing that it might disappear down the drain hole, my dad took a swift step forward to plug it with his foot. Both feet slipped forward in the mud, his back hitting the basin's concrete edge.

My dad couldn't move his arms, and my mom couldn't hear his call for help, she said. When she did, she couldn't get him out and called a neighbor. The neighbor came but couldn't lift my dad because of his own bad shoulder. My mom finally called a friend, who got my dad out of his predicament. And since the local doctor was unavailable, an ambulance took him to the emergency ward, the same place where Juliette went for her treatments.

I kept a passive face as I listened to my mom's lengthy and animated explanations, walking away so Juliette couldn't hear.

Luckily, my mom, who tends to dramatize trivial things, usually shows strength in real drama. Naturally, I tend to react the same way. My dad was in good hands, she said, there was nothing I could do but to come when I could take them home.

I tried to stay casual as I informed Juliette that I had to leave early, but from her stare, I knew I had to explain.

For both of us, it was an unfortunate reminder of my mom's irritation when I spent time with Juliette during my visits to France. This time, even Juliette's circumstances weren't facilitating our time together. It saddened me to see the resigned expression on my friend's face.

Juliette then bought a few groceries and kept disappearing in search of soy yogurts, as she explained it. She was again giving great attention to her surroundings, her face reflecting her mind, nagging thoughts likely reminding her that she'd never come here again either.

I tried not to rush her, but I felt pulled in two directions.

During the drive back to her house, we talked about my parents, who both had cancer over three decades ago (colon for my mom, and my dad was left with one kidney). They celebrated their sixty-third anniversary, enjoying each other's company in their old age, in their own home, and surrounded by family and friends. Juliette commented on how lucky they were to have each other.

Like many people of their generation, my parents were affected by World War II, yet they didn't suffer the horrible loss of loved ones—at least not physically—as so many of the French and allies' families did. They worked hard and were blessed with a good life. I felt guilty about leaving Juliette early, but my place was then with them.

Nothing felt right when we said goodbye, not even the gratification from our errands.

Juliette walked outside with me and then asked for a short lift to her community mailboxes. We hugged and kissed goodbye. Yes, I would call her. Yes, she would think of getting help at home after her chemotherapy treatments. Yes, our last moments together felt hurried. We hugged again and I cringed when she got out of the car, tearing up as I watched her in the rearview mirror. She was looking at me slowly driving away.

Would we see each other again? I am sure it was on her mind too.

My new mission as soon as I merged onto the main road was to get to the hospital as quickly as I safely could. Fortunately, driving through the border between France and Switzerland can be as quick as driving through the green light of an intersection; no one must stop anymore.

Switzerland is not a member of the EEA—the European Economic Area, formerly known as the EEC—but is a member of the Schengen agreement that abolished border controls. As of 2023, the citizens of twenty-seven countries benefit from the freedom to travel, live, or work in any of the member states, which is most of Western Europe.

I don't agree with this open border agreement, but on that day, I appreciated not having to stop to show my passport and say I had no goods to declare. I had another problem, though.

Radio waves don't stop at the border either, so the French and Swiss mobile telephone networks interfere with one another, something that infuriated Juliette. I couldn't get my mom on her flip phone.

When my parents finally appeared in the hospital lobby, my dad was in a wheelchair pushed by my mom, pale but smiling when he saw me. He would be in pain for a few days but had no broken bones. I again felt guilty that I was elsewhere in their time of need.

This ended the day of our last outing. Juliette snapping about the jacket reminded me of our past disagreements, of her adamant way of refuting my opinion, sometimes. Yet if I hadn't met her, who could have been enough of a friend to always say it as it is?

CHAPTER 10

A Pause for Thoughts

My friendship with Juliette strived despite distance and decades. What was always important to me was that she understood the disconnection I felt from living in a foreign country. That disconnection due to separation is not only physical, but also emotional; and complicated. Juliette knew what it was like to expatriate, although her experience had been different than mine.

She left for the United States as a young woman and returned to France as a wife and mother, along with the family she created abroad. And even when her youngest daughter moved there as an unattached young woman, Juliette was still anchored in her homeland during that separation. It wasn't so for me.

I left with my family while the rest of it and my friends stayed behind. Such a separation happened again when Jim retired, and we moved to *his* homeland—Canada—our children stayed in the United States.

As a result, I had to learn to share the joyful celebrations of my French family from a distance, but the feeling of exclusion has always been worse after someone dies. I only feel the real loss on my next visit—the person is no longer there. By then, everyone else has moved on with their grief—with the unspoken obligation for me to move on, too. It is as if a kind of time distortion postpones the grief until the physical distance closes, and only then does the emotional disconnection come into balance. Only thereafter can I move on.

It would take a few years to process the loss of my friend. Since moving to the United States in 1985, and then to Canada in 2002, I was no longer accustomed to Juliette's physical presence in my life, but I needed time to adjust to her perpetual absence. I was even shocked, sometimes, when something reminded me that she was gone.

For Juliette, this disconnection was so much deeper after the loss of her daughter—which I'll share later—so much deeper than mine ever was. She lost a child. She then did her best to stay physically connected to her American granddaughters with yearly visits, but whatever she did felt like it could never be enough. *This* is what distance does. In that sense, and despite our different circumstances, I feel that way too.

Juliette and I both experienced separation from family, and grieving from a distance, but unlike her, I have always had a support system.

I stay in touch through my Sunday phone calls to my parents and communicate with my *mother* by iPad—my dad worked on a computer as big as a room and could never wrap his mind around technology shrinking to the size of microchips.

It was difficult to stay connected when we moved to the United States, in the mid-eighties. On the one hand, international calls were costly and reserved for special occasions; but on the other hand, finding a letter in the mailbox was a real thrill. Today, technology helps soothe the separation.

Circumstances have often reminded me of how expatriation

and foreign exposure have changed the way I relate to my homeland, family, and friends. We all changed, but what has changed me the most is my immersion into cultures other than mine. Living abroad demands an open mind.

I first learned this as a student among other foreign students in England and Germany. We all had to adjust to a new way of life while intermingling our cultural values and beliefs. It wasn't so common in the late sixties and early seventies.

Befriending foreign students exposed the need to understand what's *external* to us so we can understand what's *internal*. In other words, I only understood my Frenchness after exposing it to 'other *nesses*.' And my occasional puzzlement over someone else's thoughts and habits was reciprocal. Our differences taught us tolerance and in return, we all gained enriching insights into other cultures.

In California, I adjusted to a culture of contradictions, in 1985. The lifestyle was conveniently modern but surprisingly unsophisticated.

It was extraordinary to me that a 'garburator' processed food waste in the sink to simplify cleaning, and that a refrigerator also dispensed ice cubes and crushed ice. But I was also dumbfounded by the hair salon I visited for the first time in Danville—the small country town that anchored the upscale housing development where we moved to.

I wondered whether I had stepped into the wrong place: the hefty dark wood furniture was more akin to those of the saloons I saw in American movies. I also discovered that blow-drying and styling didn't follow a shampoo and haircut. "Nobody does that, *here*." Really? I noticed the inflection, my accent implying that I was evidently not from *here*. On that very hot and dry summer day, I found myself on the street like a fish out of water, my hair frizzing up by the nanosecond. At least I wasn't going to meet someone I knew, which was also Juliette's comment when I told her the story. Overall, newcomers and old-timers of that charming town were courteous and simply curious about each other.

During my visits to France, I have also been meeting with my friend Marianne. Moving away to America would emphasize traits of her personality that I might never have noticed had I still lived in France.

The weekend in the mountains—with her and Jean-Paul, and Juliette and Dimitri—seems to have happened a lifetime ago, and for the most part, it did.

Marianne has been in my life in France for an even longer time than Juliette has. Yet we have less in common than I do with Juliette.

I always thought of her as being chauvinistic, but she'd retort she is simply fond of French culture, while feeling like a European citizen; even if, a priori, she isn't of a cosmopolitan mind. For this reason, Marianne knows many of the beautiful places in France. She is not a musician but learned to understand music thanks to her jazz-specialist late husband. She listens to music whereas I tend to hear it more than I listen. She likes thought-provoking, character-centred films, novels, and theatre—her son is a stage and screen actor. She also creates delicate crafts for which I have neither knack nor patience.

By contrast, Juliette had been an expat, married a foreigner, worked in an international environment, and spent time with her American family. She could relate to my challenges as an expatriate.

Overall, their differences may explain why my two friends never sought each other's company, not even in my presence. Maybe they were too alike. Marianne is now the only friend who always says it as she sees it.

My disconnection from my homeland is also due to the changes in the community where I grew up, not only in population growth but also in culture.

The village where I was born hasn't changed much in appearance but the forty-seven nationalities for six thousand inhabitants had an impact. Years ago, it blew my mind to hear mostly foreign languages as I picked up my niece from kindergarten.

Most of the residents work for international organizations and international corporations in Geneva. Juliette was part of this global diaspora. Many of our friends worked for the United Nations or its agencies (the World Health Organization, International Labor Organization, World Meteorological Organization, World Organization for Intellectual Property, World Food Bank, and the International Red Cross, to name a few). Although my parents were not physicists, they worked for CERN (the European Organization for Nuclear Research—the acronym corresponds to its former name in French, *Conseil Européen pour la recherche nucléaire*).

This brings me back to Juliette's predilection for the concept of destiny. Work brought us together because we spoke English, the common language of the international workforce in Geneva, which is also how I met Marianne—at Dupont de Nemours. We would have likely never met otherwise.

CHAPTER 11
Over the Telephone

AFTER MY RETURN home to Vancouver, Juliette and I resumed our telephone conversations. One day, she surprised me with an unexpected bout of enthusiasm.

She read my stories at *Buckettripper*, the award-winning digital travel magazine I contributed to at the time—she had accessed the link below my email signature.

She particularly enjoyed those about India that reminded her of her life with Mallick, the longest and last true love of her life, as I will tell. "The stories made me travel in my mind," she said. Perhaps they let her forget for a moment that she'll never pack a suitcase and head to the airport again.

It surprised her that I hadn't talked more about my writing, not even about a two-year distance-learning course with the London School of Journalism. We always had too much to talk about during my visits and too little time for it. Besides, Juliette always had much to say about the book on copyrights that she was editing. It was less entertaining than travel, but the fact that Mallick was the author put an entertaining spin on her comments.

On good days, she even made me laugh at times, yet the grim topic of food always came up. We talked about which was digestible yet calorific enough, but other than intravenously, her body rejected nutrition, reminding her that it was failing her. I sensed the change in her mood from the throaty sound of tiredness in her voice. I often felt my head shake instinctively—the way people do when they can't stand to hear the truth.

Time seemed suspended, and yet it kept creeping forward. One day, I called her only hours after she had returned home from the hospital. She was back there the next day. She subjected herself to this back-and-forth because, as the cliché goes, "Home is where the heart is."

By December 2013, after six of the twelve chemotherapy treatments—as I remember it—she began to doubt their efficacy. For the first time, I asked whether she was scared.

Hesitating, at first, she then began with my name, in a kind but sad voice: "Marie-Claude… sometimes… I just want… to—" then she hurled, "*scream*… but if I do, I won't be able to *stop*." She lashed out at the words *scream* and *stop* as if she wanted me to feel what she felt. A legitimate and irrepressible need had just unleashed the latent anger always simmering under her skin.

It was the primitive despair of someone who had lost the most basic of needs: control over one's life. It is so for the prisoner who is tortured, for the innocent who is condemned, and for the animal at the mercy of its predator. Juliette was revolting against a cancer diagnosis with no hope of survival. Her panicked fear gave me the chills, and it still haunts me.

Christmas brought some diversion.

She spent it at home with Corinne's family and parents-in-law, plus her son and his girlfriend. A full house pushed the fear away, at least for a day. But come the New Year, her fate would be sealed. These were weighty words to attach to a new year, completely overshadowing the challenge of new resolutions.

By the early days of January 2014, her voice sounded both forced and feeble, yet conveying weary anger, if this makes sense. One day, I immediately knew she was overwhelmingly angry. I soon learned why.

During an echography the day before, Juliette complained about her sensitive, swollen belly. Perhaps the imaging technologist felt pressured to respond, but empathy wasn't on his mind that day: "Well, you better get used to it because nothing can be done, and it will be like that until the end." I gasped before I could ask whether she was sure of what he had said. She was.

"You know… it hit me hard… as if he'd slapped my face and punched my stomach… all at the same time… I couldn't breathe."

Hearing her quavering voice made me feel as if I too had been slapped. Juliette was slowly stripped of her humanity, turning into the next medical case to be archived. She broke down as soon as she was wheeled back into her room, sobbing uncontrollably, she said. The blunt certainty of her death had been driven from her physical body to her emotional core.

Juliette had no other logical question but to ask her oncologist, not as a rhetorical question this time, how much time she still had.

For her peace of mind, she should put her affairs in order. His words were all too clear. Since the diagnosis, she refused to think about this, but the signs she'd tried to ignore had caught up with her.

After that, topics of conversation that were new to both of us deepened the psychological intimacy of our friendship. She began to let her guard down.

Short indrawn breaths filled the gaps between her words as if she couldn't keep up with the pace of her emotions. "Marie-Claude… I feel… defeated."

"I know." I ached for my friend.

CHAPTER 12

A Complicated Love Story

FOR SOME TWENTY years, Mallick had Juliette's back through her difficult times, but in the last ten years or so, she carried her loneliness and fear of aging alone.

Their relationship had taken off much like an airplane heading for stormy weather. An East Indian diplomat and senior executive at an international organization, Mallick showed an interest in Juliette shortly after she became an 'international civil servant'—an employee of an international organization bound by the UN Charter.

Juliette's strategy for acceptance was an attractive look, her smarts then safeguarding that image. For most people who first met her, there was an intriguing *je ne sais quoi*—I don't know what—about her. I had concluded early on that it was due to her polite and understated sassiness paired with her endearing guarded smile. I often observed Mallick's amused attention to her. He knew how to trigger the reactions he enjoyed, and she knew how to model her attitude to his expectations. She seduced him as much as he seduced her.

She had discovered that not all men are abusive, and he found a woman who brought the alien spice of romance into his life. He was a man who saw and heard her and above all accepted her. And so, theirs was the story of two unalike people in a complex situation, in which admiration, mistrust, devotion, perspicacity, and deceit mingled into an obsessive but lasting love.

Like Pygmalion falling in love with the ivory statue he carved, Mallick became smitten with the woman he was mentoring. He won her over by challenging her intellect and appealing to her senses. But there was one problem, a major problem. He was married and Juliette knew it.

She tried to create some distance when she became aware of their mutual attraction. Much was at stake, especially her career. Yet she kept giving in, equally smitten with Mallick's exotic gallantry and kindness. Plus, Mallick was proving what he proved ever after; he never gave up.

Their convoluted situation fuelled heated disagreements offset by the magic of their cultural differences. In fact, complications began soon after the beginning of their relationship.

We had invited Juliette and Mallick to the Caper Club, a private international club for expatriates in Geneva—I was a local, but Jim was an expat.

Mallick had refused the invitation, at first, worried that they might somehow be exposed, but Juliette's insistence and excitement won him over. Animated conversations went on at our table of four couples of various nationalities, all speaking English.

After dinner, a hesitant Mallick followed Juliette onto the dance floor, a diplomatic smile on his face. He even seemed to work on his dance steps until his composure suddenly changed. Before I realized what was happening, I was dancing with him and Juliette with Jim. It wasn't the move itself that was surprising, it was the panic on Mallick's face.

Without speaking a word, he meandered us to the opposite side of the dance floor as if it were a natural move. When the music ended, he still took the time to thank me with a contrite smile and a brief bow, then sneaked away to the lobby.

A flabbergasted Juliette then informed me that a colleague was sitting two tables behind us: we needed to change our seating arrangement. It raised the eyebrows of each couple as they returned to our table, but everyone took it in stride. Juliette's ruse was to undermine any assumption in case no one noticed them sitting together but spotted them dancing. Nothing more came out of that incident, but this was their first and only appearance as a couple at such an event.

A similar incident happened in Berlin, where Juliette had accompanied Mallick on a business trip. She was touring the city when she came face-to-face with a member of their organization. And as bad luck would have it, they were staying at the same hotel. Juliette's wit quickly spun a story about a long weekend trip with her daughter, who was shopping.

Avoiding such public encounters might be how their relationship remained apparently clandestine for more than twenty years, and how Juliette kept her job. Either their affair went unnoticed, or they kept such a low profile that people could pretend they didn't know.

Through the years, though, their quasi-nonexistent social life and the problems linked to their situation led to many crises. It was all too evident to Juliette that their relationship had to end. She also had another reason. She feared loneliness in her old age; each passing year would make it more difficult to meet someone else. I often found myself involved in their crises.

After we moved from an apartment in Geneva to a house in the French countryside—large enough for our blended family—Juliette often stayed with us to escape Mallick's tenacity when she tried to end their affair.

I often threatened to hang up on his obsessive telephone calls, but he was always impervious to my rebuffs, begging me to let him talk to Juliette or convince her to go home. Even hanging up wasn't easy because of his cunning way of keeping me engaged. Two or three days later, tired of the drama and admitting that she missed him, Juliette would give in and return home. And their complicated love story would resume for a while, through stages that were either dramatic, almost peaceful, or hilarious like this one.

During one of their early separations, Juliette had invited a male acquaintance to the apartment she had recently bought. They were having a drink on her balcony when she spotted something in the tree in her line of vision. Intrigued, she scrutinized it until intuition kicked in. Her binoculars revealed a man hiding in the foliage and, upon a closer look, that it was Mallick. Furious at first, she soon found the situation hysterical. Mallick couldn't avoid her wrath the next day when he showed up for a visit and denied everything. But wary of Juliette's determination to have him tell the truth, he confessed, laughing it off as a game.

Mallick also tried his best to prove himself if not worthy of their relationship at least useful as a partner. One of his tour de force—it means a *show of strength* and sounds more expressive in French—happened shortly after he lived mostly at Juliette's place, at around the same time. He had decided to vacuum Juliette's apartment while she was out, something he had never done in his life. Juliette laughed herself to tears as she recounted Mallick's explanations of what followed.

At first, he said he couldn't find the vacuum cleaner power button and opened the bag compartment instead. What happened next, neither he nor Juliette could figure out, but at some point, the bag escaped and took off like a deflating balloon spitting lint and breadcrumbs all over the room. Juliette found Mallick in a panicked cleaning mode, sweating like a rock star, and sheepish like a dog that just wolfed down the sandwich on the kitchen counter.

Such performances irritated her, but they made good stories. Domestic tasks were foreign to Mallick, who grew up with servants and still had a butler at his Geneva apartment.

Of course, his situation—not hers since she was free—meant that he often had to lie. He didn't want to upset Juliette with the truth, but his lies never fooled her.

When Mallick informed her of a business trip, she often discovered that there was no flight to that destination, neither at that time nor on that day. When it was a trip to London or New Delhi, she knew he was joining his wife—unless his wife was temporarily staying in Geneva, in which case he suddenly had frequent 'business dinners.'

Juliette made good use of her natural perspicacity to expose his lies, becoming her *own* private investigator. Confronted upon his return, Mallick would come up with a far-fetched story that seemed too absurd to invent, yet he stated these fabrications with conviction.

Juliette always retaliated with an all-out contempt, scolding him with fury, if not passion. But she never got through to him the way she intended because he always laughed. After all, she was the only woman who ever dared to treat him that way. But for Juliette, it was a reminder of their wrongdoing. For this reason, she often admonished him to either get a divorce or leave her alone. He would have none of it.

Mallick and his wife had two children, a son who lived in Geneva, and a daughter who had died of cancer a few years before Mallick and Juliette met. For a time, Juliette accepted his refusal to divorce because of his wife's broken heart. But after two decades, she was losing patience. Mallick appealed to her compassion when she threatened to call his wife. Juliette understood, even before she, too, had lost a daughter. And so, from one ultimatum to the next, their complicated love story continued.

If it's true that diplomacy is the art of using negotiation techniques to have someone let you have your way, then Mallick was a master of that art. He knew how to turn a bad situation into an acceptable one. And when Juliette was skeptical—which was most of the time—she often pretended she wasn't, too exhausted to keep bickering. Her confrontations were always bolder than Mallick's, who usually gave in as a compromise for the life he couldn't give her.

Despite their conflicts, there were long truces during which they were devoted to each other, appreciating each other's intellect and culture. What's more, beyond the romance that bound them, there was also the exotic physical attraction. One could extrapolate the Indian sexual culture—from the erotic sculptures seen on temples and in the reproduction of ancient documents. On our trip to India and tour of Rajasthan, a guide explained that these sculptures appear only on the outside walls of temples as a reminder that the inside must be free of lust. As for ancient documents, sex is therein considered spiritual and not hedonistic. We took his word for it.

Back to Juliette's relationship with Mallick.

Jim and I often enjoyed convivial evenings with them, Juliette cooking a hearty meal paired with the appropriate wine. She familiarized herself with enology and kept a well-stocked wine refrigerator in her garage. She and Jim often talked wine while Mallick and I sipped it sparingly. Born a Muslim, Mallick indulged only in a few sips, and despite my French genes, I am not much of a drinker either. Mallick and Jim got along, appreciating that their fields of executive work were at opposite poles. Jim dealt with international business and Mallick with international politics.

Mallick also took great pleasure in entertaining us with jokes about diplomats, some more offensive than others, like this example of, well… a logical fallacy in a syllogism: "If a diplomat says *yes*, he means *maybe*; if a diplomat says *maybe*, he means *no*; and if a diplomat says *no*, then he is no diplomat. If a lady says *no*, she means *maybe*; if a lady says *maybe*, she means *yes*; and if a lady says *yes*, then she is no lady." This provocative joke highlights that such disrespect at the expense of women is unacceptable today, but it illustrates Mallick's strategy for argumentation.

Whether Juliette and Mallick's relationship could have evolved steadily had their circumstances changed, no one knows. Meanwhile, Juliette's derision was an engaging contrast with the apparent submissiveness of the Indian women of Mallick's generation. As was prevalent in his youth, his marriage was arranged. And as often happens with such couples, Mallick came to love his wife in his *own* way. But it was never romantic love as happens in our culture when two people fall in love freely.

Our tour of Rajasthan gave me such an insight, from an interview published in *Asian Age*—an Indian-English newspaper. According to Indian celebrities who were asked what the Taj Mahal meant to them—in 2004, India was celebrating the mausoleum's 350th anniversary—Indians are not attracted by the architectural beauty of the Taj Mahal so much as they are by its symbol of exceptional love—between the Mughal emperor and his favorite wife, who died in childbirth, and the reason he devoted his life to building a mausoleum as beautiful as their love.

At some later point in their relationship, Mallick surprised Juliette with an invitation to accompany him on his upcoming trip to India. Such risk was so inconceivable that she took it as an auspicious sign. But after they set foot in his homeland, she hardly saw him during the day and spent her nights alone in her hotel room. Her bitterness was spoiled by the luxurious accommodation and private tours Mallick organized for her enjoyment.

Why did Mallick invite her? Juliette had no answer. From my perspective, perhaps taking her to India was a promise he could keep.

CHAPTER 13

California, February 2014

In early February 2014, Juliette had an appointment with her oncologist to assess the impact of the chemotherapy treatments. An ultrasound would give the verdict, which she called *la grande inconnue*—the great unknown.

She was reading a book about Diana, Princess of Wales. Corinne gave her books on meditation, which she found 'uninviting.' She even drove to a hair salon that uses natural products but refused a haircut, not trusting that it'd be as she expected. I made her laugh as I remembered reading that for long-haired Jim Morrison—the American singer and poet—haircuts were some of the worst mistakes in his life.

I emailed her almost every day to give her something to look forward to. I wrote about insignificant daily matters. She could read these written messages as many times as she wanted. It gave us something else than her condition to talk about on the telephone.

One day, I shared that my stepdaughter moved a few minutes away from where we had lived for seventeen years—before we moved to Vancouver—and close to my son and his family. Juliette had visited us several times in California. She could imagine me going to the supermarket and remember us browsing downtown Danville.

I babbled about my first night in that house; me and boxes while my stepdaughter was on a business trip. I had no television or house phone, but a cell phone and an Internet connection through a network key, likely unfamiliar to Juliette who wasn't keen on computer technology. I even mentioned the quieting hoot of the same great horned owl I would hear most of the nights that I spent there since then.

I didn't expect a reply to my small talk, assuming she may be past that kind of diversion. But she did answer. "You are busy, and I am lonely," was her first comment. She was also doubting the benefit of chemotherapy. *J'en ai marre*—I'm fed up—she wrote in her no-nonsense signature style. She sent her *affectueux baisers*—affectionate kisses—a French term of endearment to end a letter to a family member or a close friend. I often felt like both.

It would be her last email.

She called a few days later. Cancer was progressing faster than chemotherapy, she said. I responded with an empathic moan. Symptoms don't lie.

She knew because she couldn't keep any food down and yet her belly kept swelling. She knew because she was in pain. She knew because she hardly recognized herself in the mirror. And yet she still didn't want to know.

From then on, there were often new silent gaps in our conversations. It's not that we avoided talking; there was nothing more either of us could say.

There was no point in telling her that, had the tumor been discovered when it was still contained in her pancreas, she could have been among the thirty-seven percent of patients who survived for five years; but this was 2014 and in 2023, PanCAN states that it's forty-four percent. At the time, I hadn't heard of the Whipple procedure, a complex surgery to remove the head or the whole pancreas, sometimes also a part of the small intestine, bile duct, stomach, plus the gallbladder and nearby lymph nodes. It's very complicated and risky, but it has saved lives. Perhaps it was too late for that for Juliette unless it wasn't available at the hospital, but that option was never discussed.

One day, after one of our wordless moments, she was the first to talk again. Calm, grave, and almost apologetic, she said, "It's my destiny… There is nothing we can do… I have no choice… I must accept it."

From five thousand miles away, I swallowed my tears and tried to control my ragged breathing. Was she beyond the revolt, or was she trying to convince herself? I wasn't sure. All I could say was that I admired her wisdom while sorrow burbled in my throat.

"I am going to die of… starvation." She loved to cook, and now she couldn't even eat. She mentioned euthanasia, legal in Switzerland where she was treated. The following week, she thought of stopping all treatment. Two days before she did, I received a message from Corinne.

February 7, 2014

Dear Marie-Claude,

I hope you and Jim are well. Mom is asking me to thank you for the beautiful bracelet—she loves the three colors and the very soft clothes that she couldn't try on. As you might know, she returned home the day before yesterday after receiving a different type of chemo than the last one, which didn't yield any good results. But she got so sick from that new chemo and so weak from being undernourished and lying in a hospital, she couldn't stand on her feet. After twenty-four hours, we had to take her back as an emergency. […] The question now is to decide whether chemo should be stopped, and palliative care started. Yesterday, she felt so sick and desperate she wanted to die. Enduring all of this gives her extreme anxiety […] She doesn't know that she has another tumor. […] Today, the worst of this last crisis has subsided, and she is feeling a little better, although there is never any complete relief. […] She wants you to know that from now on, you can call her in the hospital, which is the reason for me writing to you. I wanted you to know exactly what's happening even if you cannot discuss it with her. She will tell you herself. I wish I had better news.

Love to you and Jim.

Corinne

I couldn't read the email again, wanting to put aside all that it meant. I recall last September when Corinne's oncologist—the same as her mother's—explained that Juliette's body produces a type of mucus that makes chemotherapy ineffective. It seems that chemo was doomed before it even began and yet it continued.

This brought on the disturbing vision of my friend fading from life like an overexposed photograph. I couldn't think of her pain. I couldn't think of her fear either because *I* was fearful of what lay ahead.

Dear Corinne,

Thank you for your message. I called Juliette on the

day that she returned to the hospital. She felt extremely weak and feared ending up in a palliative care facility. She wants to stay home. [...] Jim and I are both very sad; it's a horrible situation for her and you all. I will try to give her comforting words, but it becomes more and more difficult. I normally go to France in June. I could come in May instead.

Love,

Marie-Claude

When I talked to Juliette, after these emails that she was unaware of, we tried to find some encouragement from her decision. No more chemotherapy meant no more nausea and perhaps eating without throwing up. She could rest and peacefully prepare for the journey of no return. But it wouldn't happen quite that way. All I could do then was support Corinne by sharing my sad perspective.

Dear Corinne,

I sent you an email earlier today before I called Juliette. It was a very sad conversation. She said she would probably not see me again. [...] I am a wreck right now. She wished I were closer. She sounded very scared, yet she had moments of incredible serenity. She talked about her destiny taking its course. I don't know what to do. I would like to have an idea of when it would be best for me to come. I wonder if talking to her doctor would help. Let me know.

Love,

Marie-Claude

That evening, and in between time zones, Corinne sent another message.

Dear Marie-Claude,

I just read your messages. You are with her all the time, with your calls and your sweet intentions. It's hard to know when the end will occur, she may live two months. [...] She is strong at times. However, she also says that she is going to die; she knows it. [...] I will not push for extra chemo; she just needs peace and enough pain relievers to go toward the Light. The Light is so bright it cannot be described. [...] I told her she was beautiful and so did my daughter. Her eyes are deep and sometimes scared, but her soul is clearing day after day. All is now a matter of fighting or letting go. It will be the case for all of us one day; the secret is to die to what you are. [...] As I once wrote in a poem for a colleague who had taken her own life: "Because life is just a passage, and you another me." Be in touch. Hugs.

Corinne

I woke up the next day, thinking of Juliette held captive by her illness. I was angry at the helplessness of the doctors, the inefficiency of therapies, the discouraging statistics, and the seeming inertia of scientific research. Research was doing what research could, but progress was too slow for those who need a cure now. Juliette's loneliness was deepening, the terminal stage of cancer isolating her no matter what her family and I could do.

She was dying. We weren't. The loss of control over her life added to her afflictions.

February 8, 2014

Dear Corinne,

Thank you for your moving words. I talked to Juliette

this morning. It was very difficult. [...] She repeated she wouldn't see me again and that her destiny was taking its course. She was still wondering whether stopping the treatment was the best decision. [...] She said she needs to feel calm, but the treatment has the opposite effect. [...] I am happy that your spirituality helps her talk about dying. [...] Hugs.

Marie-Claude

It was all going fast, too fast. On the positive side, mother and daughter could talk about death whereas even the weather could lead to disagreement before. That Corinne cultivated an interest in metaphysical matters was helpful. I hoped that the bright light that she'd described brought some peace to her mother's mind as she faced something that happens only once in anyone's life.

CHAPTER 14

The Meaning of Time

JULIETTE COULD DO nothing with her remaining time except put her life in the perspective of her past and her short future. Her present consisted of living through one day and one night and soon one moment at a time. This was on my mind when I woke up in the morning.

Since her retirement, loneliness and loss were uninvited but frequent guests. The two men she loved had betrayed her, each in his own way. They were gone; the magic of their relationship with Juliette had died before they did. Then, her relationship with her son and oldest daughter was a source of frustration, and her youngest daughter took her own life, leaving behind Juliette's then-eight-year-old twin granddaughters. And now Juliette had arrived at the end of her own life story. She felt lonely perhaps because, along Amy Tan's views in *Where the Past Begins*, loneliness is more about misunderstanding than aloneness.

Juliette's short survival time was her ultimate loss. Despite the cases of "beyond-all-odds decades-long remissions," pancreatic cancer is still uncurable, and most long-term remissions happen when it's caught early. Whether chemotherapy slowed its progression, or not, her only hope was that it would extend her life a little longer.

Time never mattered as much as it did then. It was still sort of tangible, but she would soon no longer be on its grid. As for the idiom 'buying time,' one can't buy it or extend it from one's own free will. Even 'time is money' is worthless in the face of mortality. Unlike time, money can be earned again, but death has its own agenda, and it's always free.

Time only matters when there is life.

It begins at the time of our birth and ends at the time of our death. We somewhat regulate our lifetime by the way we use it, but it still dictates our life. Even a baby's life is regulated by feeding, burping, bathing, sleeping, and playing times. Time then puts pressure on adult life with the necessity for working time, seldom balanced with leisure time.

With the evolution of our civilization, technology now controls us too. We can achieve more in a shorter time than we ever did before, yet each day unfolds like a race to meet obligations, many of which we impose on ourselves. Ironically, we are called *the human race*, which now sounds like a subliminal message that man's destiny is to race to the end of life. I can still choose to avoid falling into the trap of time, but Juliette no longer can. Still, it's increasingly difficult to avoid the technology trap.

This brings to my mind a course in mythology and a Sumerian philosopher—I forgot his name and couldn't track that textbook. Around 2000 BCE (Before the Christian Era), this Sumerian philosopher observed that humanity declined as technology advanced. Even the land of Sumer experienced what we do now.

Located between the Euphrates and Tigris Rivers—in what is southern Iraq today—this first organized civilization was the cradle of ours. Sumerians invented the wheel, canal irrigation, basic mathematics, and among other things… writing. Even the world's first credited author was Sumerian; a woman who signed her name *Henheduanna* to a collection of poems.

One can argue the immense differences between Sumerian technology and ours and be baffled by the philosopher's claim—that the invention of the wheel affected the way people lived. Yet his observation still makes sense.

A distant precursor to robotic mechanization, the wheel put some laborers out of work as mass production did in our civilization. And like in the ancient land of Sumer, the disappearance of many of our traditional trades has affected the way people interact.

Sophisticated technology enables us to maximize the use of time yet fails to improve our lives at all levels. Electronic devices transformed human relationships into virtual connections. We text instead of talk. This shift affects the way we live to the point that some fear that our dependence on electronics may be initiating the decline of our human sensibilities, and perhaps that of our intellect as we increasingly rely on devices. Scientists agree that technology in its various applications contributes to stress, psychosomatic illnesses, and desensitization.

The argument goes even further.

Overexposure to violence—in films and video games—is seen as the link to that desensitization. The American Academy of Pediatrics warned that children may become desensitized to violence to the point of growing up thinking that violence is acceptable. It again makes sense. After all, at the other end of the spectrum, even a beautiful view becomes normal when we see it every day.

Ironically, the Sumerians initiated our race with time when they divided each hour into sixty minutes. In the end, our perception of time is what we want it to be, to enjoy, or to waste, or to miss the point, as in my take on the story of the fisherman and the businessman.

A successful businessman goes fishing, once a year. He sets up his fancy gear by a river when he sees a man upstream. When he meets him, he notices that the man is poor. He is disheveled, his clothes are worn, and there is no fancy fly for his old rod. The businessman points out that having a job would improve his life; he could then afford a vacation, nice fishing gear, and enjoy good times. The man remains silent, his eyes set on his fishing rod until he says, "I fish any day I want to and catch fish for dinner every time. Why would I change anything?"

For Juliette, the abnegation of choice was total. She lost control of how to spend her days and when her time would end.

CHAPTER 15

The Valentine's Day Gift

I HAD FIRST planned to go to France in June, then decided on May. Yet Juliette was still asking and Jim still urging me not to wait. But going sooner felt like I'd take away any hope that she'd still be alive in three or four months. I finally admitted my denial.

Jim called Juliette on Valentine's Day to say he had a gift for her. That gift was *me* coming sooner.

The next day, her faint voice answered the phone and got immediately livelier. In four days, I'd fly to Geneva directly from San Francisco—where we were still visiting our children and grandchildren—and stay in France for two weeks.

Two days later, I received another Facebook message from Corinne.

February 17, 2014

Dear Marie-Claude,

She will be so happy to see you. What you chose to do is wonderful. This time, we must absolutely see each other. My uncle will come on his way to the south of France with his family, and I am not sure when. You are right, she needs company and love, that's all. I am looking forward to seeing you, but I must warn you that she has slipped deeper into the illness. It's odd to see her like that but for me, she will always be beautiful. Affectionately,

Corinne

I pondered Corinne's warning. My friend had "slipped deeper into the illness." I also wondered what our first impression of each other would be, after so many years. Corinne likely knew I was aware of her stormy relationship with her mother, a situation that puzzled me since I only knew one side of the story. But from her thoughtful emails, I sensed we'd get along.

And that's how, six months after Juliette's diagnosis, on this day in February 2014, I am trying to get over a stubborn case of bronchitis, resting on a sofa at my stepdaughter's house, and looking at nature out the window. So much happened since I first learned of Juliette's illness in August 2013.

I am also preparing myself mentally to 'accompany' my friend because this is what she asked. I forget most of what else she said. Her words were so explicit I broke down and stopped listening. But I heard enough to know what she meant. She wouldn't be alive in June, or in May, and probably not in April either.

With Corinne's email lingering on my mind, I get up from the sofa, wrap a throw over my shoulders, and step outside.

The sun has softened the air into a mild winter afternoon. I take deep breaths as I look at the towering redwoods, inhaling their balsamic whiffs. The trees might be fifty years old, and still in infancy considering that in old-growth forests specimens reach thousands of years. Endemic to the West Coast, redwoods are amazing examples of survival.

Whereas humans often fail to meet life expectancy, nature organically engineered redwood trees to survive dry California summer days and years of droughts—thanks to the nightly fog. Never mind that groundwater collected by their roots can't reach their top, they collect it from the sky. With time, the oldest specimens rely on what has become a spongey canopy, an ecosystem that doesn't exist in new-growth forests. Nature prepares for adversity better than humans do.

My mind wanders until my gardener's eyes take over my stepdaughter's new backyard and land on leggy bushes in need of pruning and yellowing lemon trees in need of fertilizing. All living things are connected and when taken out of their natural environment they need help.

I envision the blooms that would brighten the garden. Then I see the geraniums left by the previous owners. Ah… a pleased sigh escapes from my heavy heart as I snap the first of the faded flowers. And I think of my friend's garden left to fend for itself.

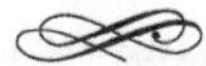

I GOT OVER my bronchitis just in time before my trip; thyme infusions with lemon and honey, vitamin C, zinc, and other supplements were maybe less of a cure than rest and patience. That Juliette can't count on anything to feel at least a little better belittles complaining about a visit to the dental hygienist, a Pap test, or a colonoscopy.

Still, I am frustrated as I pack for my trip to Geneva; I have clothes for winter in California, not for Switzerland. Then I remember: I am going there as my husband's Valentine's gift to my dying friend. This puts my frustration in perspective.

As I fold clothes and wrap shoes, my thoughts take me back to last year.

Juliette was talking about her first paracentesis, a procedure that drains the abnormal fluid—called ascites—which fills the peritoneal cavity and causes the belly to swell. Her mind wrestled with that duality. On the one hand, she felt better after the liquid was gone. On the other hand, she abhorred the thirty-minute procedure; a long needle inserted two inches into her belly, under local anesthesia, draws out what she knows is a liquid of cancerous cells.

I also remember my last visit, over October and November of 2013. It was disheartening that the little food she ate no longer nourished her body. She was pleased to still have hair but coloring it didn't matter anymore.

At the time, and as it would happen, I feared that Juliette might have only a few months to live. Her oncologist had been as indirect as the rhetorical question she asked—advising her not to think about it and focus on the treatment instead. But he did warn her about the challenging treatment and insisted she stay positive. Juliette accepted her doctor's faint encouragement, but cancer would have the last word.

After I finish packing, I call Juliette.

She says the disease is taking hold of her body, that something is pushing everything up and there is a burning acidity in her throat. She might not have enough time to put her affairs in order. She also worries about her daughter.

Corinne is exhausted after six months of her mother's illness, her unsettled family life, her job, and her long commute every day. I also know from Corinne's messages that bridging the resentment gap between them was necessary and redemptive, but also emotionally draining. From Juliette's deep worry for her daughter, I hear a positive shift in their relationship.

I ask Juliette what I can do to help when I get there. She doesn't hesitate. I haven't given it much thought and will do anything, but her answer takes me off guard. I'll organize her funeral.

I am unprepared to hear about something that usually happens after a person has died. I hold my breath at the mind-blowing thought of discussing it with her, and that planning her funeral will be the focus of our last days together. When I hang up, I feel numb.

CHAPTER 16
Transitions

TODAY IS FEBRUARY 17, 2014. I am on a late flight for my fourteen-hour trip from Vancouver to Geneva via London. This refuge in the sky puts me in a meditative state. I relax and doze on and off. I am in a bubble of sorts, and it deepens my sense of physical and mental space.

In this flying vehicle, transporting me through the atmospheric void some 35,000 feet above North America, across the Atlantic Ocean, and to Europe, and despite some three hundred other passengers on board, I feel isolated. A sense of transition, of passage, and it's not from displacing from one continent to another: the New and the Old World combine to form a global entity. It's about feeling drawn to the ephemeral vision of an afterlife as I gaze at the free-formed white clouds that amble in the blue sky. After all, people always look up to the sky when they think of Heaven.

Life in this temporary biosphere relies on technology and physics, eluding gravity, and connecting only indirectly with people on the ground. Nothing could prevent this aircraft from nosediving or spiraling into a crash from a mechanical failure or other unforeseen interference.

It's like the mental passage from free will to fatalism. It's both liberating and sequestering. Air travel gives me the clearest thoughts as if they were free from the pull of subjectivity. As if my life were cut loose, or on *pause*. In turn, this odd sense of relinquishing control gives me peace.

After landing at Heathrow Airport, deplaning turns into the usual pantomime. Life unfolds like an obstacle course.

Passengers bolt from their seats as soon as the seat belt signal dings. They grab their carry-on bags from the overhead compartments and inevitably someone is jabbed. They turn their cell phones on while waiting for the gangway, then race to their connecting flight as if they are about to miss it, or to the baggage claim as if their suitcase might evaporate. Never mind that most of them will end up in a queue at passport control and security screening.

I imagine the viewers of a futuristic History Channel, bewildered by the burdens of the travelers of the past.

The contents of pockets, shoes, belts, and jackets land in one or two bins, and carry-on bags in another. Electronics get out of their cases and into yet another bin. By then, these devices will of course look antiquated. Ah, let's not forget the medications in plastic bags and the plastic water bottles tossed in plastic trash cans; never mind that this plastic will be a bane for generations to come. And while all bins then disappear on a conveyor belt, passengers walk barefoot or sock-clad through the metal detector. And then all steps are repeated, only in reverse.

I have the recommended two-hour overlay, but today it's barely enough, even using the priority line. I don't mind the rush—it keeps me focused. But when the airplane takes off for the last leg of my trip, anxiety grips my chest. My mind is fast rolling again.

On that late sunny afternoon flight, I gaze at the French part of the Jura Mountains, in the direction of Geneva. This mountain range was the natural, and logical, border between France and Switzerland until that border was pushed back and forth over centuries of warfare.

In the foothills, the familiar string of French villages and towns face the distant snow-covered peaks of the Alps and their crowning Mont Blanc. The Rhône River has left Geneva to meander through a valley of agricultural land, a patchwork of colors recurring with the seasons.

After a smooth landing, we roll at great speed by the Swiss Airlines airplanes parked in front of their hangars. The familiar logo of the Swiss flag, red with a white cross at its center, was square trimmed to fit the tail fin, and replaced the Swissair design. This new rendition of the flag had raised controversy in this country of almost nine million citizens who vote on everything. In the end, maiming the flag was deemed a business decision unrelated to Swiss governance.

When the airplane stops, the excitement of arriving home fills me up. Greater Geneva is one of my homes, and having an enduring attachment to each one makes me somewhat of a global citizen. My paternal family lives here, as do friends—one of whom is waiting for me to 'accompany' her to the end of her life. I am on an unfamiliar and sad mission, but my attention quickly returns to practical matters.

Like other European airports, Geneva International Airport has its annoyances: deplaning through a steep mobile staircase rain or shine, walking onto the tarmac to a satellite terminal, and hoisting carry-ons to clear the steps down another steep staircase. And, after a long walk, surprisingly outdated luggage carts await.

I explain to a frustrated passenger that he must first withdraw money from the ATM, and then use the bill-to-coin changer to get the Swiss two-franc-coin that will release a cart. His frown says it all. Unlike the eight-dollar cart in San Francisco, at least in Geneva you get your two francs back—upon returning the cart to a concession. Better yet, handy luggage carts are free in Vancouver. As for the free one-hour Wi-Fi connection, you have three cumbersome options. The easiest one is at the departure level, not the arrival: a bright pink machine—somewhat like an antique mailbox—will scan your boarding pass and give you the access code. Don't bother expecting a timely code by phone for the other option.

A family friend meets me at the arrival level. Having met Juliette, she offers her heartfelt words of encouragement. Driving by the hospital reminds me that Corinne prepared me for the change in my friend. Talking over the phone was all about the voice, but this ultimate reunion will have no such filter.

I hear Juliette's sigh of relief when I call her after settling down with my parents. I'll see her mid-morning tomorrow. She tells me I am her angel. I tear up, not sure I am that angel. Hearing her voice reminds me that she'll rely on me, and trust me, in the next two weeks. And that's when I also remember a lesson that I learned many years ago: I must be in *her conversation*, and for this, at some point, I must ask, *"Are you afraid of dying?"* I learned it from Heidi—an extended family member—when I visited her in the hospital in Bern, where her brain tumor proved to be inoperable.

I remember with fondness boarding with her parents while

attending school in German-speaking Switzerland. Every morning, I awoke to the sound of Heidi's practice of the composition for piano of the theme from *Love Story*—the blockbuster movie starring Ali MacGraw and Ryan O'Neal. After seeing the film, we talked about it in a café, our teary eyes gazing into our cups of hot chocolate. We were young and couldn't have imagined that she'd die at the age of thirty-nine.

And so, we talked about that brain tumor, the chemotherapy that took her hair and made her sick, and her young children.

When there was not much else to say, awkwardness came between us, and *the question* blurted out of my mouth before I had time to think: "Are you afraid of dying?" I remember holding my breath, shocked by what I'd just said, but Heidi looked at me with a sad smile of acknowledgment.

"You are the first to ask… Everyone else is afraid to talk about it."

I don't remember whether she replied in German or French—I wasn't so fluent in German anymore—but I know what she said.

Only after her eager answer to my daring question were we able to truly connect. Not avoiding the subject of dying had put me in *her conversation*. People kept telling her not to give up, she would beat *this*. They knew the truth, but it made them feel better to say *that*.

She thanked me for having the courage to ask. But it wasn't courage. It was an instinctive, somewhat impulsive, but heartfelt and desperate urge to connect, to offer compassion. As if I could somehow carry a minute part of her burden.

Conversely, and despite their good intentions, her visitors made her feel "more alone than if they hadn't come." She felt misunderstood, isolated, and worse, she felt lied to. Was she afraid of dying? The answer wasn't really needed but the question was.

By the next summer, she was receiving palliative care at her parents' home. She couldn't open her eyes, but she acknowledged my presence with a faint smile. Silently, I promised never to forget *the question.* She taught me that unless we are in the dying person's *conversation*, we let a wall rise. Truth invites closeness, and it's what that person needs. It won't happen without it.

Since then, the *Love Story* soundtrack doesn't bring the movie to my mind but the memory of a lesson about the end of living and the beginning of dying. The two are but a moment apart, one revealing the sacredness of its miracle and the other the mystery of its finality.

Heidi's passing is another example of distance creating disconnection. I heard the sad news from my mother, during a regular phone conversation, two weeks or so after Heidi died—the formal announcement came later. No one told me because everyone thought I heard it from someone else. I was sad, but I also felt left out, even if it was unintentional.

My then seventeen-year-old son felt that disconnection too, at first refraining from showing sorrow over the loss of his beloved godmother, his father's sister. He couldn't share his sadness with his Swiss family. There was nothing to witness. We were *here*, and it happened *there.*

As I lie in bed on my first night back in France, I know what Juliette will need from me and it's not hope.

CHAPTER 17

Geneva, February 2014

THE NEXT DAY, I rise early because of the time difference and chat with my parents, catching up on French and family news over breakfast. Then I drive to Geneva to visit Juliette in the hospital, for the first time since last October.

On the way there, I try to prepare myself. I find I can't. I am eager to see her but apprehensive of the moment our eyes will meet.

I park my car and walk toward the lobby's automatic door, an imaginary balloon inflating in my throat. My breathing is shallow. I know the reunion will be difficult.

Inside the lobby, small groups occupy the sitting area. I imagine that the smiling ones are taking turns visiting new parents and their babies, but I also notice the gloomy expressions of those who are stooped in armchairs, waiting perhaps for a loved one to survive a risky surgery.

The receptionist greets me with a smile and gives me Juliette's room number.

"It's on the second floor to the left, close to the elevator," she says. I prefer to take the stairs, then absent-mindedly I go right instead of left and don't find her room. I keep walking, looking at the numbers on the doors until I have made an entire loop back to the stairs, and come upon her room, to the left of the elevator as the receptionist said. Juliette would have reminded me that I have a terrible sense of direction.

This detour seems to have happened for a reason. I am now ready to see Juliette.

After a courtesy knock, I walk in and find the bed closest to the door empty; she must be in the one by the window. Then I see her. I assume it's her as I take hesitant steps forward.

Juliette looks at me with a tight-lipped smile as I take in the shock of discovering what my beautiful friend has become. She is even thinner than I imagined. Her eyes have further receded. Her cheeks have sunk, guarded by a protruding upper jaw. I immediately see the imprint of death on her etiolated face.

I kiss her forehead then bring a chair close to the bed, trying to smile a little. I don't know what to say. I am relieved when she talks first, slower than she used to.

"You know… Jim's call on Valentine's Day… it meant a lot more than I can say."

She received it as if it were proof of our friendship. Never mind an intercontinental trip, but a short visit, a phone call, a card, or flowers, *these* are our last chances to show we care. Many years ago, a younger me hadn't realized this until it was too late. Death hadn't waited for my goodwill.

I wondered what my last days with Juliette would be like. It's the first day of my two-week visit and I already have a hard time. I try to let my instinct guide me, but my thoughts bump into one another, and like in a maze they come to dead ends.

It's hard to begin a conversation with a close friend who is terminally ill. I am sitting at her bedside feeling as if I am with someone I just met. A mental fog numbs me, and yet it looks like

I am listening to her intently. I am struggling in the presence of the new *her* and grateful when a health care professional brings a welcome diversion. He is a physiotherapist.

Does Juliette want to walk today? Given her physical state, will her frail body carry her? I wonder, and I am shocked when she says, *yes*.

The man helps her get on her feet and then off she goes, out of the room, holding on to the intravenous drip walker, the physiotherapist at her side, and me in tow. From her unexpected brisk pace, I question the physiotherapist with a look.

"Juliette has been quite a fast walker." He guessed my silent question.

"Only people who have time to waste walk slowly," she fires back.

We walk by a couple sitting in the open lounge of the floor, and I catch their grave, furtive looks at Juliette, who looks straight ahead, marching on at the beat of our small talk. The image of a brave soldier heading for the front enters my mind until she suddenly has enough, stops, and turns around. Like Tom Hanks in *Forrest Gump*. This defiant stroll has visibly exhausted her. We slowly return to her room where she nearly collapses before a nurse helps her lie in bed. We don't talk until she smiles at me with a hint of pride, evidently expecting a comment.

"You still have your hair!" Still shocked, that's all I say.

"Yes… but… you know… I have been walking… almost every day." She is still catching her breath and I realize too late that she expected praise or some kind of validation for her effort.

I have already failed her.

I then watch her pat the top of her head and then the sides of her face. "Oh, my hair… It's stringy… I don't brush it… I'm afraid it will all fall out if I do… but… it's better than no hair at all—no?"

"Yes…" I reply, somewhat unsure of this. But I see in her eyes that it's a little victory over her failing body. "You're wearing the fluffy socks I sent you. You know they contain a moisturizer, right?"

"Yes, and I love them *so-oo* much. They feel *so-oo* soft on my skin. I'm sorry I can't wear the lovely lounge clothes and pajamas you sent. I can't bear anything around my belly." Then she explains what I already know.

She can't keep any food down. She enjoys smelling, tasting, chewing, and swallowing it, but she pays for what is hardly an indulgence. Eating causes stomach pain, nausea, and vomiting. Intravenous feeding makes up for her body's inability to process food.

"I feel I have begun to die from hunger." The intolerable fact flattens her voice. I move closer and bring my hand to her cheek. She holds it there, tightly. Our faces almost touch. We look into each other's eyes in silence. Then she watches me cry as if my tears assuage her own emotional pain.

Late at night, I lie in bed, unable to sleep. Her ghostly smile haunts me as soon as I close my eyes. I try to remember what else we talked about but only remember what I saw. The bald patch at the back of her head as she walked, the matted hair clinging to the side of her neck like the long earflaps of a Peruvian hat, her loose watch sliding to her elbow when she raised her hand. *This* is what I saw, and no treatment could have prevented this wretchedness because there is no cure.

It angers me that we found ways to send a man to the moon

half a century ago and then improved the space exploration of our solar system by leaps and bounds, while in the meantime on Earth, the pancreatic cancer detection method remained inadequate during that same half-century.

It's frustrating too that, according to *Public Health Reports*, it takes an average of seventeen years for fourteen percent of clinical research studies to be integrated into physicians' practice. What about the remainder of these discoveries, you may ask? They never translate into practice.

Before falling asleep, I think of Juliette's frail body, of her sharp mind that carried us both this afternoon. She is still the incorrigible talker. I am still the listener.

CHAPTER 18

Reconnecting with Corinne

JULIETTE SAID I would 'accompany her to the end of [her] life.' On my first visit yesterday, I didn't want to rush into what it would involve. And today, I don't know how to begin that conversation about funeral arrangements. She must be reading my mind, bringing it up. First on her list is to get a plot at the cemetery of her village. I don't flinch.

"It's a nice cemetery. I like that it's on a hill," she says.

I know exactly where it is. The cemetery is on one side of Saint-Brice Church, a typical setting in France. Juliette doesn't go to church but must have checked it out. She might have stood there, hoping for some encouraging yet elusive insights. She might even have approved of the recent restoration of the cut-stone walls, the off-white grout matching the stone in a *cerusing* effect—when wood is rubbed with a white pigment.

My attention returns to her, speaking in truncated sentences, and somewhat annoyed.

"I asked Corinne. To call the *mairie* [the city hall]. To buy a plot. I don't know. If she did. She still hasn't called. So. I still don't know."

"You said Corinne is coming later—she'll likely tell you then."

Discussing this over the telephone would be difficult, although face-to-face won't be easier. My guess is that Corinne juggles her time between work, family, and her mother. Besides, it requires a daunting question. One must buy a concession—the 'right to use a plot for burial purposes for a pre-determined time.' Asking her mother whether she wants her grave for thirty or ninety-nine years, or in perpetuity, won't be easy.

Juliette interrupts my silent quandary.

She wants a granite monument with an integrated planter—she's thought about this. Blooming plants last longer in soil than in pots. I recognize her straight-to-the-point way of dealing with things. Her son likes nature and will take on the ritual of caring for her grave. I agree with a series of nods; I am taking mental notes of her last wishes. She reiterates she wants a church service. The funds in her checking account will cover the expenses related to her funeral… She speaks as if she is thinking aloud, or to make sure it will happen.

"Juliette, don't you think you should involve your children?"

"I want to get as much done as possible, with your help. Corinne is so busy… I can tell she struggles. I asked her to take care of the plot because—" She hesitates, and I can't imagine what she is going to say next. "I don't know how long it takes… I don't know when… I'll need it." Then she adds that her son is too devastated to help.

To understand Juliette, one must also know about her children.

Her son developed schizophrenia in his late teens. The condition affects the way one thinks, feels, and acts. It can generate strange ideas, depression, paranoia, addiction, and the hearing of voices. Juliette has been supporting him because of his difficulties in staying employed. The last times I saw him, he was kind and withdrawn, but his instability frustrated Juliette.

As for her oldest daughter, Juliette often complained about her indifference, and belligerence too.

Juliette shared such feelings with angry impatience. As if she was reliving what caused them and couldn't wait to vent. She resented that her daughter didn't include her more in her family life, for example. When she took each teenage grandchild to visit Paris where she was born, her grandson told her he asked his mother why they didn't see *Lili*—Juliette's nickname as a grandmother—more often. Amid the family rifts, her grandchildren's affection was of great comfort.

I haven't seen Corinne since she, her brother, and her late sister attended Ecolint, the French abbreviation for *École Internationale*.

The private, Geneva-based international school was founded in service of the League of Nations, in 1924. I am familiar with its standardized education system that prepared my oldest stepdaughter for the International Baccalaureate—an entry-level diploma to worldwide universities.

Corinne and her siblings transferred as teenagers from a French high school to the Ecolint English immersion program. Corinne would go on to work for a United Nations agency and go on a six-month mission to Vietnam.

It's my second visit to Juliette on this trip and 'the Corinne' I meet today is now a middle-aged woman.

My first impression of Juliette's daughter is that she stands tall and lean like her father and has his high cheekbones. Her hair is short, unlike her mother's. She wears classic dress pants and a tone-on-tone blouse. Her necklace and bracelet show that she likes ethnic-style jewelry.

We kiss three times, one cheek after the other—a regional custom for salutation. We had connected through writing and talking over the telephone, but to see her again after decades is like meeting her for the first time. I needed her guidance when I was far away, and I now need her presence to help me support Juliette.

After getting reacquainted, we get organized. Corinne will visit her mother during her lunch breaks and take extra time off when needed. I will come every afternoon. I know we'll make a good team to 'accompany' Juliette.

CHAPTER 19
The Secret

I CALL JULIETTE every morning to let her know when I'll be there that day and every evening to wish her a restful night. It's a comforting routine for both of us. I don't visit on the weekend; her family does.

I didn't visit either when, one day, her friend—I forgot her name—flew from Milan.

We briefly met years ago when Juliette moved in with her—after running away from another violent dispute with Dimitri—and until she got a job and could afford to rent a flat. Her friend had eventually moved to Italy and was making a one-day trip to say goodbye, which meant a lot to Juliette.

On another day, out of the blue, Juliette talks about her father. I still know nothing about him except that he died many years ago. I don't know what suddenly prompted her to say something like: "He has meant nothing to me for a long time," and in a tone of voice that was shocking.

When she pauses, I implicitly wait to hear why, but she hesitates. She then looks down at her hands clasped on her lap and blurts out that when she told him *his salesman abused her*, he slapped her hard and called her a liar.

I don't remember the exact verb she used, but despite the

blunt accusation, she didn't say *raped*. Regardless, a sexual violation is an indelible imprint on the psyche.

When I ask whether her mother knew about this, Juliette says she saw the whole scene—her complaining and her father slapping her—but she never spoke a word. And it was never mentioned again. Juliette doesn't elaborate, but from the way she looks away, her bent arms half raised in front of her and palms toward me, she is unwilling to say more.

I am shocked by her revelation, which immediately sheds some light on my friend's enigmatic persona and her unpredictable reactions sometimes. I am sad that it happened but also feel more than a twinge of hurt. Why did Juliette wait so many years to tell me this whereas I shared my own trauma, years ago? How old was she when this happened? Did it have anything to do with her move to California in the sixties? Questions race through my mind, but she is silencing me. Besides, this is not the time to upset her.

That she waited so long to confide in me makes me wonder how many little girls will grow into young women with tangled selves and how many have already gone through life with a broken sense of trust in others, and themselves, too. And do not know why.

Accusations should never be dismissed—even a child's reticence toward a family member or a 'trusted' friend. That child may have a reason to feel uncomfortable.

According to thehotline.org, an average of more than one out of three women and one out of four men will experience rape, physical violence, or stalking by an intimate partner—in the United States. In most cases, the perpetrators first gained the trust of their victims.

Abuse is an injury to the mind that leads to trauma. Sometimes it blurs the memory of it, but it will always warp the ability to trust. Because a past trauma lingers in the emotional side of the brain as a 'present' that never leaves. Even reckoned with, it's never forgotten. That Juliette refrained from sharing this may explain the latent rage beneath her skin, and her dismissive ways sometimes.

Trauma is like a bulb planted upside down. The plant will twist to grow toward the sun, and from that invisible entanglement, a stunted bloom will barely conceal that something went wrong underground. Unless trauma—no matter the type—has been shared, faced, and reckoned with, it retains its destructive power.

Then we both remain silent. What else is there to say? Only she, knows.

CHAPTER 20

A False Alarm

THE NEXT MORNING, I wake up to the roar of cars passing by as if everyone drives to work at the same time, which of course they do, usually to Geneva. Jet-lagged, I had only fallen asleep a few hours earlier, but it must be seven o'clock since I can also hear my parents.

I know they are up from the doors that my dad bangs closed, which irritates my mom who trained herself not to make noise when he slept part of the day after working a night shift.

I let them have breakfast and watch the news on the small television in the kitchen. They always have *brioche* with unsalted butter and a generous amount of my mom's often homemade jam. They gave up coffee for a substitute dissolved in hot water and sweetened with nothing less than two heaping spoons of sugar. It's a lot, but my dad justifies it, half-jokingly, by saying—translated word for word from French—*sugar builds muscle*. Evidently, with a few shortcuts: sugar provides the energy necessary to build muscle but has no nutritional value.

I am grateful to still have my parents, which also allows me to enjoy this house. My dad built it in the sixties, with the help of friends—a favor he returned when they built their own homes.

I like the familiar coziness of my small bedroom, upstairs in the back of the house, and was quite upset when my parents replaced the faded Laura Ashley wallpaper with a white, blinding imitation of textured plaster. "It makes the room look bigger," my dad said.

Things have changed around us too. Housing developments encroached on the farmland, so I no longer hear cowbells. My dad resigned himself, proud to point to a partial view of the Alps and 'Napoleon's hat.' His passion for history has nothing to do with the local nickname given to a configuration of peaks that emulates the iconic bicorne hat.

I am also fond of the view of the *château* (the castle)—a unique depression in the topography of that precise part of the Jura Mountains. But most baffling is the alien screeching sound of a macaw, sunning itself in the small garden of a nearby low-rise apartment building. I could also go on about the nightly whiffs of marijuana that ascend to my open window in the summertime, from the house closest to us. They don't even help my jet-lagged nights.

This morning, I will take my mom on errands after giving Juliette my usual morning call. When I do, I am surprised that the nurse answers the telephone and says Juliette can't take my call.

I have breakfast, planning to call again before lunch.

As I often do, I enjoy plain yogurt from the sheep's milk of a local producer, and Wasa crackers—that my dad calls *cardboard bread*—yet delicious with butter and my favorite honey—from a beekeeper relative.

Today, I get my dad's smile of approval when I don't hesitate between croissants and cardboard bread. I drink herbal tea, although giving up caffeine made no difference to my jittery menopausal episodes. At least it gave me an excuse to avoid Juliette's coffee—brewed French style, in a percolator that turns it unpalatably bitter. That's how it's served in most French restaurants, with sugar, although even Parisians have developed a taste for Starbucks.

Two hours later, I am rushing to the hospital.

Juliette was in a total state of panic when I called the second time. When I first called, the nurse was informing her of her impending transfer to a palliative care clinic. Stunned by this sudden turn of events, I listen.

Juliette is no longer entitled to a hospital bed because she is no longer receiving treatment. She must leave the familiar environment of the hospital where the nursing staff has been *so-oo* supportive. She'll be sent away to a village outside Geneva and will feel disconnected. Corinne won't have time to visit during her lunch break, and the traffic through Geneva will be horrendous at the end of her workday.

Juliette dreaded palliative care, rejecting all mention of it. She doesn't say, but had she known this, she may have decided to continue with chemotherapy.

This also complicates my situation. Instead of ten minutes, it will take me an hour to drive to the clinic, and two at times of heavy traffic. I am also in France to visit my elderly parents and already feel conflicted. I quickly decide: Juliette is the priority.

There won't be a *next time*.

When I arrive at the hospital, Juliette is discussing with the nurse whether to relieve the pressure in her belly by draining it one last time. Paracentesis won't be available at the clinic because—in her case—palliative care means no treatment.

Juliette is upset by this procedure, a reminder that her belly 'is full of cancer.' From what I understand, food fuels pain, exacerbating her failing digestive system, even if she vomits it back up. There is no good choice because not eating starves her emotionally too. In the end, she accepts the paracentesis to satisfy her yearning for food, a little longer.

"I need something that gives me… you know… a little pleasure."

"Yes… besides, *you* have the right to decide."

We don't say anything else.

As 'luck' would have it, her transfer gets postponed several times, but we don't talk about it. Every morning that she can stay becomes a good day until it dawns on her to ask the nurses why her transfer keeps getting postponed. No one 'knows.'

No one says that she'll go when someone has died.

CHAPTER 21

Of Father and Mother

THE RISING SUN blurs the grayness of the winter morning. Buds add a pop of lime green on the plum tree in my parents' courtyard. The tree is as old as the house—more than half a century. A black fungus darkens its trunk, yet the espaliered branches will soon bear bundles of pink flowers.

In recent years, my dad has been tempted to cut down the tree, but my mom keeps watch; the trained horizontal branches screen the veranda from the road. Besides, "Doesn't the tree still bloom?" My dad only smiles at her rhetorical question.

Meanwhile, he obsessively controls the fungal spread with an otherwise harmful chemical. His resolute argument is: "Without chemicals, the world would starve."

He defends their use by referring to the fifties, when fertilizers and pesticides boosted farmers' production in Europe, improving a standard of living degraded by two world wars.

Recently, however, and after the subject kept appearing in the science magazines he subscribes to, he acknowledged the unintended consequences of these chemicals: they poison soil, water, food, and all living things. Still, until effective eco-friendly solutions replace these chemicals, he has a point.

Meanwhile, thanks to my mom's vigilance, and likely to the

harmful chemical, the old plum tree still stands. My dad admits that the tree still has plenty of life. Like him, its limbs are aging, and its insides are slowing, but it still shows off its might. Nobody knows how long the remission will last, but the tree will die when the fungus wins.

Juliette's body began to die when no one could see it and even *she* couldn't feel it. When cancer revealed itself as a mask of faint shadows on her face, malignant cells had already overtaken her body. The spread of the fungus on the plum tree has been in remission for more than a decade, but such a long remission happens only to a minority of stage IV pancreatic cancer patients.

When I call Juliette, we almost take for granted that it's another lucky day. We don't talk about the looming transfer from fear it might end the postponement. Today, though, I find her upset when I arrive in her room, and it has nothing to do with her impending transfer.

She is expecting a telephone call from a family law attorney. Her brother will be the executor of her estate, handling her mother's as well as hers, she says. I am confused. Have I forgotten that Juliette's mother died? Perhaps she forgot to tell me.

From what I know of their mutual animosity, and his lack of support in the past, I am also taken aback by her brother's offer to be the executor. Corinne would later deny her uncle's offer, and her mother asking him angered her.

The fact that Juliette's mother died may have been lost by the detached way in which she shares even significant information, sometimes. I may not have understood this. I do, however, begin to add things up about their relationship.

Her mother failed Juliette after she accused her father's

salesman of abuse. She never called Juliette on her birthday although Juliette always called on hers. She criticized or contradicted Juliette on everything as if she took pleasure in angering her only daughter. She even gave money to Sophie—Juliette's youngest daughter—when she was in rehab in Paris, despite Juliette's fear that it would tempt her to buy drugs. Worse still, she held Juliette responsible for Sophie's addiction, and indirectly for her death. A tragedy I will share later.

One day, she informed Juliette that she had disowned her. Juliette's resentment was still raw months later. It had nothing to do with the money and everything to do with her mother's deliberate intention to hurt her. Of this, Juliette was sure.

Then Juliette's mother struck one last time before she died: saying Juliette was "old enough to be sick." With this last blow, I could tell from Juliette's reaction that she'd lost any compassion she may still have had for her mother. She let her mother 'go' before her mother even 'went.'

Later, after reading one of Corinne's emails again, I came upon the fact that she and her brother were going to their grandmother's funeral in Paris. Juliette was already sick then.

Juliette suspected that her mother may have been jealous, although in a convoluted way.

When Juliette and her family moved from California to Paris, they lived with Dimitri's parents for a while. Then after her father-in-law died, her mother-in-law moved in with them. By then they lived in France, near the Swiss border, in the house that remained the family home until Dimitri moved away. Juliette often talked about the tension from Dimitri's ever-present mother interloping in their marriage. Plus, Dimitri's work as an interpreter demanded flexible hours. Juliette was on her own much of the time, raising three young children and caring for an elderly woman who spoke only Russian.

Perhaps Juliette's mother resented their apparent closeness, albeit imposed. But as I would later hear, there was more to her mother's life than Juliette shared.

Back to the attorney.

Juliette is irritated that the attorney keeps her waiting inconsiderately whereas she has no time to waste, as she puts it. And as if she needed a release, she suddenly rages about seeing her mother on television. I don't know what triggered this, but I am about to hear another vivid story.

Juliette was watching the news when her mother supposedly appeared in a segment about care facilities for the elderly in the Parisian area.

"Imagine my surprise when I saw her!" she says, anger rousing a bout of energy. "She was sitting sideways… I immediately recognized her. She was wearing the same blouse… as when I visited her last year."

"Are you sure it was your mother?" I am still baffled by the turn of her conversation.

"I'm sure… I even saw the same segment on another television channel. There she was… from the back this time… with the same blouse. I saw her with my own eyes!"

From Juliette's agitation, I can tell that nothing could convince her of the contrary.

Juliette's need for attention and her reveling in stories of happenstance often made me wonder whether some truly happened. Yet I often got the evidence that even the most mind-boggling ones did.

Juliette looks at my reaction to the television story, the expression on her face emphasizing what the tone of her voice expressed: bitterness, resentment, and defiance.

"Can you believe it? My mother managed to nag at me all the way to my deathbed."

She says this in one breath, then exhales a puffing sigh of bitterness. I don't question what she says she saw. Her mother is dead, but she could still have appeared in a documentary. Or did a woman who resembled her mother bring back Juliette's resentment? I'll never know, but it reminded me of Paul Coelho's words. In *The Alchemist,* he refers to the idea that coincidence doesn't exist in this world.

Perhaps Juliette's imagination helps her exorcise the pain her mother caused for so long. Meanwhile, I am once more the dumbfounded audience of Juliette's dramatic storytelling. But more than resentment, I again hear hate in her voice.

Juliette cringed at the thought of dying before her mother and although her mother died three or four months before she did, it didn't appease her.

Why did Juliette not find peace from this? She never said and I never asked. She might have answered that *her mother waited for her to be ill, to die*. Unless she felt robbed of attending her funeral.

Whatever the reason, Juliette never got closure if not meaning on such miserable feelings.

CHAPTER 22
Past and Present

BOTH OUR PASTS are at a standstill in the back of our minds, but my present unfolds toward the future whereas Juliette's is bound to the walls of a Swiss hospital, closing in on her. Whatever happened or is happening or will happen matters less and less; she has little if any control over it.

Such thoughts are on my mind as I leave my parents' house and work out that I'll arrive there in fifteen minutes, thanks to the opening of the border.

It's a confusing geographic dynamic that *Pays de Gex* is now an official transnational suburb of Greater Geneva, yet even before this, Geneva was an essential part of our lives; going *en ville* (downtown) meant going to Geneva, not to the nearest French city.

I sometimes hesitated when a customs officer asked whether I'd bought more than the duty-free allowance, which was never by much. Juliette was bolder than me, often using her magnetic charm to plead for an officer's indulgence. Since the opening of the borders, commuters and travelers are expected to operate under the honor system, but officers are rarely present, so locals tend to cheat a little. The real problem, though, is the lack of control over illegal goods and undesirable people.

Years ago, Juliette was unusually silent upon hearing that a thief had come into our bedroom suite in the middle of the night, in Southern Spain. The next morning, the officer just shrugged when we filed the police report: by then the stolen goods had likely changed hands several times; they were either on their way to France, and from there anywhere throughout Western Europe, or on a boat to Morocco. Unlike the USA, the European Union is a multinational entity. Imagine driving freely between the member states of the USMCA agreement—formerly known as NAFTA—the United States, Mexico, and Canada!

Today, I am surprised that Swiss police are present at the checkpoint. They must be looking for a specific vehicle, so they wave me through before I even stop.

Past the border, I immediately come upon the CERN and the distinctive wooden Globe of Science and Innovation, a symbol of planet Earth, and the interpretive center for visitors of the fundamental nuclear research that is done here. The road then slices the agricultural part of the municipality of Meyrin and, a few minutes later, I am parking at Hôpital de la Tour.

When I walk into Juliette's room, Corinne is taking notes over the telephone and points to a chair, indicating that I should stay. When the telephone conversation ends, she gives me a quick hug and rushes back to work.

The family law attorney was dictating the text for the power of attorney to Juliette's brother. Juliette is restless and impatient to take care of today's task, so we do.

She reads each word aloud before writing it. I secure the page on the overbed table, her unsure hand penning each letter until she signs the document. She asks me to mail one copy to her brother and one to the attorney, which the receptionist helps me do. She then asks me to place the original in the inside pocket of her purse—as was agreed upon. When it's done, her shoulders rise then she releases a deep sigh. She is grateful for the resolution of a matter that had angered her the day before.

I understand right then that she won't be at peace until everything is taken care of. It also comes to my mind that I never met Juliette's brother.

She was so bitter when neither he nor his family called after Sophie died, and yet, he was Juliette's liaison when Sophie was in rehab in Paris. Then Sophie moved to the United States, where she died tragically some ten years later.

Juliette attributed his silence to the influence of his wife, who thought of herself as the perfect mother, a status Juliette felt she could never match. Yet the siblings' relationship somewhat mellowed after the family gathered for the ninety-fifth birthday of their mother, four years or so before mother and daughter would die. It raised Juliette's spirits to feel somewhat acknowledged by her family, but that truce wouldn't last.

Since their mother's apartment in a Provencal village needed renovation, and brother and wife planned on doing the work themselves, Juliette insisted on doing her part. What happened next is another example of Juliette's knack for creating a dramatic story out of a simple spat.

All went well until they disagreed over the color of the tiles. Her sister-in-law chose a light ocher that Juliette was adamant would turn too yellow. As their voices began to rise, Juliette's brother slammed the door, leaving the women in their disagreement. Only later would I hear from Corinne that, at a loss to get her way, her aunt threw a tool—I forgot what kind—at Juliette. I couldn't help chuckling from envisioning the scene that made

Juliette give in. And as her keen eye for decoration would have it, the light ocher was too yellow.

As usual, when telling a story, Juliette stretched it with every detail. This often made me want to tell her: *please, summarize!* But there was no telling Juliette to keep things brief.

When she recounted a situation, she relived it with the same feelings. As if she needed to set the record straight, even if it was for no one else but herself. She never mentioned that failed ocher tiled floor again. That color, however, kept appearing like a sign.

Juliette has drifted into sleep, exhausted from having written the power of attorney. When she wakes up, I confirm again, and again, that I did mail copies of the document and that the original is in the side pocket of her handbag. I imagine that putting her affairs in order is like her last *raison d'être*, her last *reason to be* in this life. Each confirmation validates her accomplishment and calms the sense of urgency in her mind.

CHAPTER 23

The Difficult Questions

A CONVERSATION WITH Juliette is never simple in her hopeless situation. I didn't anticipate how complicated it would get after suggesting that she talk to a counselor or a priest; they could help her in ways that I can't. But Juliette objects almost in the same breath as she reiterates her wish for a religious funeral.

"What happens… after death?" she sort of pleads.

I am speechless since it's the first question of that kind. I can't help looking away, even if her stare is softer. My mind begins to race like cars on a track, too fast to let me focus.

"Uh… I've read theories that… resonated with me, but… no one knows for sure." When our eyes meet again, I can tell she expects more than my evasive answer. I stumble onward.

"All I know is what I've heard… or read… and what I think too. Death means different things to different people… you know… because, well… God doesn't mean the same thing to all people. It's complicated… We see this world… and we try to understand it… but we can't sense it completely… Something makes us feel there is more to it." My monologue is punctuated with short silences, giving time for my thoughts to stay on track.

I pause to allow her to say something, but she doesn't.

"For some people… God is the religious figure… for others… God is Mother Nature… and for others still, God is a concept, a 'presence—'" my index fingers make air quotes "—within themselves. It's not that they pretend to be God, but that's the way they feel a divine connection." I hope she'll ask another question or change the subject, but she lies in her bed still and silent, and ready to hear more.

"Who knows… death might even have something to do with some extraterrestrial power!" I say this as a diversion, but she doesn't fall for it. I feel pressed to continue. "People who think scientifically say the brain stops like the switch of an electric outlet that's turned off… that there is nothing more. Others get a sense of the unknown, of a mysterious afterlife. And still, others believe in heavenly life. Since it can't be proven, that's why it's called *faith*."

I want to end this complicated conversation about theories that I sense but never had to express before.

As I talk and she stares, a detached look on her face, it dawns on me that she may only want to hear my voice and not so much my answer to her question. Perhaps she expects me to tell her what *I* believe.

And I feel so unprepared.

"You've heard of people who died medically, and then their hearts started to beat again." She nods at my rhetorical question. "Some say they saw a beautiful white light… they felt surrounded with love and peace. They felt guided and welcome, uh… perhaps to what that *more* might be. But… neuroscientists gave a medical explanation for that light." Juliette still says nothing. "It's comforting, though, to know that this loving white light felt, uh… godly."

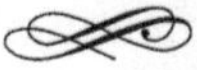

AT THE TIME, I didn't know that people of various faiths have different visions: Hindus see Krishna or blue-armed gods, and Muslims see Muhammad. For sure, Juliette would have asked what neuroscientists have to say about that.

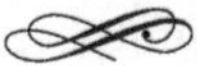

I LEAVE IT at that, relieved to have articulated a matter as physical and yet as abstract as death. Then I wait for a guiding cue.

"Could you prop up my pillows?"

Quiet and pensive Juliette looks outside the window. She always sees the same apartment buildings under a sunny, cloudy, or rainy sky. Today, it's under the early dusk of the last winter days. Soon, streetlights and people's apartments will silently glow in the darkness. Juliette doesn't hear life outside the hospital's walls. None of this brings the vision of an inviting white light filled with godly love. Still, it gives me a glimmer of hope that she got a glance of it. But if she did, I ruin it with another theory; namely, she might see in the afterlife people she knew in her earthly life.

"*Ah, non alors*! (Ah, absolutely not!) There are people I really don't want to see again!"

I can't help chuckling, but I don't only hear cynicism in this uncharted conversation for both of us, I see it on her face. She did *not* intend to be facetious. I try to calm her indignation with a compassionate smile. I have upset her and must find a way to make up for it.

Before her illness, I often took advantage of my chatty friend's hesitations to speak, but words are failing me now. Under her interrogative stare, I again stumble onward.

"Some people say they have 'contacts'—" my index fingers make air quotes again "—with the afterlife. They say that '*there*'—" air quotes again "—love is of another dimension. It's universal, without judgment, unconditional." Words come out of my mouth as if someone whispered them in my ear.

I worry that I am entangling myself in some psychic philosophy. I wish I were better prepared for this. I haven't studied the Bible to cite it, and my years of catechism in France less than inspired me. Still, it wouldn't appease Juliette who refuses to talk to a priest. Besides, no one came back from *there* to tell us how it is, and a religious leap of faith never was in Juliette's life repertoire.

"Well… I doubt that heaven exists…" She lets her comment hang, then lowers her eyes to her hands arched on her swollen belly. Unlike an expectant mother connecting with her unborn child, Juliette seems to console her body for the cancer she is gestating.

"But… what if hell does?" Her stare goes right through me.

Ah, how shall I answer that question? Bizarrely, Descartes comes to my rescue, *I think, therefore I am*. I am not sure how the French philosopher's quote is relevant to that very moment, but right now, at least it gives me a shot at some logic.

"Aha… if you're afraid that hell might exist, you can't exclude that heaven might too. You can't have one without the other, you know!" I take her hand and wait for her reaction. I feel the palpable emotion in her pressing fingers as she lowers her eyes to our joined hands.

"I haven't been an evil person, but—" she sighs "—I have regrets. I am afraid my life hasn't been—" she hesitates, looking for a word "—exemplary."

I place my other hand over hers, hoping some soulful thought will help me appease what sounds like a confession. I know almost everything about Juliette's life since we met, and much of what happened before that. At least I think I do. I know my friend as a good person who was hurt in too many ways.

"Juliette… you have regrets because you learned from your life. You wouldn't have regrets otherwise. If your regrets are sincere and you ask for forgiveness… uh… to the whole universe… since you don't want to ask a priest… then you'll be able to let them go."

She listens intently, silently.

"Many selfless, innocent, and good people go too soon. Some say it's God's plan… but others say that a good God wouldn't let it happen. Then some must face their prejudices because they turned back against them, sort of like a boomerang… They too must learn." I can tell from the spark in her eyes that I have struck a chord.

"Aah… then you mean that I am a faster learner than you?" Her wit is back—a good sign.

The tease in her eyes enlivens her face and lifts both our hearts. Then she releases my hand and turns to the window again, looking up at the sky. And from my lightened heart, I imagine celestial thoughts freely swaying in her mind like flags in the wind…

And from this, a gentle quietness descends upon us.

The four o'clock snack interrupts our implied need for silence. She declines any beverage or cookies but insists I have some herbal infusion: "because it's what you like." I oblige, grateful for this moment of normalcy.

I sip the warm, soothing verbena brew, my playful smile suggesting I admire her courage, her candor, and the humor that often empowers her. Cancer may be holding her body prisoner, its rapacious grasp tightening day after day, but it doesn't stop her from being funny at times.

"I'm going to write a book about you," I hear myself say on the spur of the moment.

"You will." She says this as if it were a fact. I am shocked. Then she asks why.

"Because… you have such a graceful way of dealing with all *this*…" My arms open in an all-encompassing gesture. "I'm learning so much from you… it could help others too… perhaps two friends like us." I can't bring myself to say that it could answer the question, *what is it like when your friend is dying?* "Besides, some of your stories are truly worth telling, you know." I notice the contented smile of someone who, against all odds, scored two points at once.

A book! Later that night, the thought spins in my mind.

I remember my childhood friend's father telling me I should become a writer; I was thirteen years old and sending expressive letters at his long-term care facility. It took me a long time to get back to writing.

I was working on a fictional story when this promise of a book burst out of my mouth. More than fulfilling a promise, it would also give a sort of continuance to Juliette's life; defer the unavoidable fading memory of her.

As it would happen, the idea of that book was a blur for months on end. Still, *I am going to write a book about you* was no shallow promise. I knew it would be a consuming task that wouldn't leave me alone until I fulfilled it.

Pancreatic cancer then became the enabler for this book. Unbeknownst to me, though, writing it took me on a journey more reflective than I could have imagined.

CHAPTER 24

An Unusual Store

CORINNE AND I have an appointment at a funeral home. I imagine Juliette's reasons for demanding that's what we must do next. She had a lot of time to think that she could still weigh the *now* but not so much the *then*. We can go today, or we could go in three days, but *then* is not guaranteed. She needs the peace of mind that all is ready when the time comes.

When Juliette first asked me to help with her funeral arrangements, she didn't want to know any of the details. Bizarrely, she rejected the very thoughts of what she wanted the most.

In a far-fetched comparison, it's like the mixed emotions I'd have if I wanted to parachute from an airplane but resisted the thought of it. Thinking about it would help me prepare, but my mind wouldn't want to anticipate the fear of it.

A few years later, I was reminded of Juliette's dilemma because of my mom.

My parents and I were at the cemetery on All Saints Day, placing the traditional pots of chrysanthemums on our relatives' graves.

My mom had been saying for a few years that she wanted the monument on their grave-in-waiting to be installed, that it would appease her. Knowing my mom, it was more about ensuring that it'd be to her liking, and it was okay with me although it wasn't with my dad. "Look at this sad slab of cement," she said that day as we walked by it. "I should have brought more chrysanthemums." Perhaps my mom was less joking than trying to soften my dad into agreeing with her wishes. Perhaps it would indeed soothe her—and help appease her fear of the unavoidable transition to what Juliette calls *the unknown*.

Corinne and I are ready to go, but a sort of embarrassment hinders our departure. I fidget until I find something to say.

"Corinne let's take my car… it will give you a break from driving." I say this as if we were going on a casual errand. "Juliette, we'll be back in two hours or less." And I say that as I give her a furtive look before opening the door, taking in all at once her sadness, helplessness, resignation, and incredulity.

I feel guilty that I can't wait to get out of the room, down the stairs, through the front door, can't wait to take that usual deep breath and let go of the awkwardness. The brisk air clears my mind and invigorates my body. I glance at Corinne. She looks grave and tired. We don't speak. We don't need to. She is going to buy her mother's casket, although her mother still lives. Grief hasn't blanked her mind yet. The thought is raw, unprocessed, real, yet numbing.

On the way to the funeral home, we are both still silent. I keep my eyes on the road while Corinne looks sideways, mostly at freshly plowed fields. It's still winter, and the sky is of that crisp blue that suggests it's cold outside. I drive over a former rail track, its typical guard house now expanded into someone's home. When the line was still active, the *barrier guard*, as he was called, activated the red warning lights, and manually lowered the barrier to stop traffic. It used to be an event that we, kids, enjoyed watching even after it was electrified. Today, some villages are now converting these train tracks into pedestrian and bike lanes. Change is part of life.

Halfway to our destination, we begin to chitchat in desperate need of diversion.

"You know, some of Juliette's traits make me cringe," Corinne suddenly blurts out.

I am shocked that she refers to her mother by name and baffled by the hostile comment. As if being away from her dying mother has brought back the resentment she felt before she became ill.

"My mother always talks too much… and she takes over conversations… to draw attention to herself." There is reasonable truth in Corinne's complaint, but I cringe at her bluntness under such circumstances.

I get more tense as she continues to criticize her mother, who "fills her house with stuff that lacks spirituality," as a way "to fill her empty life."

Very upset, I nevertheless bite my tongue.

The newscaster on the car radio fills the silence with words that I don't listen to. I sort of gaze at the road in front of us. It's the first time I've heard Corinne share a reason for resenting her mother and it's quite untimely. I avoid responding and then wait before asking whether the twins will come from the United States soon or wait for Juliette's funeral. She doesn't know.

The conversation then turns to Sophie's lost life and her complaints about their mother.

"What do you mean… Sophie always felt worse after your

mother's visits?" Her new accusation overpowers my ability to keep my mouth shut.

"She made my sister feel lower than dirt. She always felt she judged the way she lived her life." I huff a loud sigh of impatience but can't respond; we are arriving at the funeral home.

It's my first experience of it, and now I am not only apprehensive I am also troubled.

I park in front of a detached house with a large sign that reads *pompes funèbres* (literally, *funerary processions*). The curtained windows of the upper floor indicate that it's also someone's home. At ground level, a front window displays memorial statues, plaques in concrete or bronze, and ceramic flower arrangements.

After Corinne rings the bell, the door opens to a woman dressed in a black blazer, gray skirt, and white blouse. The funeral home director invites us inside.

I look around the unusual 'store' as she points to the chairs at a table and to 'the catalog of services and prices.' The very thought of a funeral *catalog* tarnishes what I see as a solemn mission. I am also shocked at the astronomical cost of a 'funeral package.' Then our task becomes complicated as soon as the woman asks questions.

Juliette will be buried in France after dying in Switzerland. The process for the repatriation of the body depends on the geographical location of her death: the hospital or the palliative care clinic. In the latter case, a sealed zinc casket will transport the body to a mortuary chapel in Geneva, where it will then be placed in the wood casket…

The woman turns the terminology of her industry into a flat delivery of standard sentences. It feels odd to decide on something that hasn't happened yet. Besides, I resent that my friend be already referred to as *the body*. As for Corinne, she looks horrified at the thought of her lifeless mother sealed in a metal box. From her love of nature and interest in Eastern philosophy, she struggles with the necessity of a *zinc* casket.

"It's the law!" the woman retorts. Then she excuses herself—called to the office next door. Corinne and I whisper. Would Juliette approve of being so 'preserved'? I dread having to discuss this with her.

As I would hear later from Corinne who contacted another funeral home, the obligation to a zinc casket didn't fit the situation. Evidently, dealing with a funeral home is an emotional process for loved ones and a business for the undertakers. The wrong decision can lead to dramatic consequences as in my aunt's case. I don't recall sharing this story with Juliette, perhaps because this drama didn't yield any memorable wittiness.

On the funeral day, my cousins had gone to the Swiss mortuary chapel to witness the sealing of the allegedly compulsory zinc casket, but it was already sealed and none of them gave that permission. Panic quickly replaced consternation; another casket was released that morning, and now no one knew for sure who was in the remaining one. To make matters worse, the seal could only be broken across the border, at a French mortuary facility. Worst still, only an accredited official could reopen it, and in the presence of someone other than a family member—to identify the body. As a result, my aunt's service began two hours late, and many attendees had left. And yet none of this should have happened since the law didn't apply.

Back to the current funeral home.

We follow the woman into a room with caskets displayed on

slanted shelves along the walls. I identify those in pinewood from their knots and the citrusy scent I become aware of. Unfinished pine coffins are the cheapest, usually bought for cremations although "it's not mandatory, but most people do anyway," the woman says.

I learn the difference between *cercueil* (cheaper, tapered, or six-sided, often referred to as *coffins* in America) and *coffre* (expensive, rectangular, and called *caskets*). Glossy rosewood is the priciest, and in between are various finishes of oak. Deciding on style, handles, crosses, linings, and embellishments is overwhelming. The funeral industry calls them personalization products, memorialization products, and other print products.

I think of all the people who did this yesterday, tomorrow others will, today it's us. Juliette is likely imagining what we are doing here. Tears blur my vision. Corinne wraps her arm around my shoulders. I didn't think of offering her that comfort.

One year ago, Juliette and I talked about our lives, trips, gardens, clothes, and hair. Today, I am looking at caskets for her funeral while she consciously awaits death. When I look at a lined lid, it looks back as the ultimate closure on life. Whether it's lined or not.

It dawns on me that dealing with a funeral home is part of the grieving process.

Because of circumstances, I seldom attended funerals in France. In America, I attended those of my husband's parents and aunt, and of a few acquaintances.

I haven't seen many dead people either. The first was our old neighbor, when my brother and I were kids; his familiar long nose sticking up from his supine body. Later, I was briefly shaken by the open casket of a friend's father in his military uniform, after walking from the back of the church to pay my respects. And I saw Jean-Paul in the Swiss mortuary chapel.

Today, I am fighting with the thought of my friend laying in one.

CHAPTER 25

The Conversation

I DON'T REMEMBER driving from the funeral home, preoccupied with all that our mission entailed. Corinne was silent, gazing at the farmland along the way. At the hospital, it's the busiest time of day for visitors. I don't mind having to look for a parking space; I am apprehensive about returning to Juliette's room.

When we walk in, she turns her head toward us, and I wish she were asleep to give us time to get composure.

We look at her observing us as we approach her bed. Her face is unreadable. I immediately feel a wider divide than when we left. Reality likely settled deeper into her mind, as it did in mine and likely in Corinne's too.

Selecting her casket affirmed the unraveling of her life, affirmed her destiny. It's no longer in the vague, it's in the short future, not quite now yet, but it's coming. With awkwardness, we resume our presence at her side.

Corinne gently asks her mother how she is doing while we take too much time removing our coats and staring at the wall hangers. She seems to wait for Juliette to say something, something that will ease the uncomfortable transition, but Juliette doesn't.

When I finally face her, I have no choice but to speak. I read in her eyes the expectation of an answer. I feel as if Corinne and I are two kids who must confess to some mischief. She waits for us to talk, *us* the bearers of 'news.' Somewhat blank-minded I stand at the foot of her bed for what seems like long minutes.

"So?" she says.

So? What does she mean? What shall we say, exactly?

I hear Corinne's deep inhalation and feel pressed to say something, anything. "It's done--you don't have to worry about it anymore."

Juliette hesitates, then asks what choices we made.

We stand as still as actors eager to hear the director shout 'Action!' or 'Cut!' But this is no make-believe scene. I don't know what to say, how much to say, or how to say it. I don't know whether Juliette is trying to fill the silence or needs a description of the casket, lining, and other trimmings. Did she change her mind about not wanting to know the details? I feel pressed to reply.

"It's simple and classy." Surprised by my words, I still hope I don't have to elaborate.

"What color did you choose… for the lining?" She could be talking about a new dress.

"White." Corinne's one-word answer fills only an instant.

Juliette notices our uneasiness and stops asking.

We have no choice but to answer her questions, volunteering information, though, doesn't come naturally. It crosses my mind that she might be teasing us to relieve the palpable tension.

This situation brings on the wish that death wasn't so taboo in our culture. That it would be an accepted part of life as it is in other cultures, some even 'feeding' their dead, changing their clothes… The vision might be creepy, but then it wouldn't be so hard and feel so wrong to talk to someone about the casket they'll soon inhabit.

"What were the other colors?" From her lighter tone of voice, she may be enjoying holding the reins of a situation that is entirely about her.

Corinne looks at her mother, ready to say something, but no sound emerges. Then she looks my way, and I look at Juliette just as she looks at me. This is when Heidi dying of a brain tumor crosses my mind. It reminds me that we must be in Juliette's *conversation*.

"Uh… the choices were… uh… light blue, but you don't like blue." Pleased that I remember this, she replies with a nod.

"Or pink."

She frowns.

"Then, there was gray—"

She interrupts: "No! It would be too depressing."

"We didn't think you'd like mauve." I am easing into *her conversation*.

She rolls her eyes. "*Oh là là, non!* It reminds me of my mother's old housecoat."

I smile, but I sense that something about the color bothers her.

"You don't want white?"

"No, it's not that… You chose well."

Corinne stares at her mother, guessing there is more to it, too.

"It's just that… white won't go with what I want to wear for my last… uh… dress-up."

Our gasp brings an amused reaction to her face.

"Juliette! Only you would think of it this way." I smile the way I would at a naughty child.

"Well, we don't know how they dress on the other side." I take this last comment as her way to end this very unusual conversation.

But it's not over.

"I would like my photograph on the headstone. I've noticed that people do that now." She hadn't mentioned this before, so she'd obviously thought about it while we were away.

I visualize the framed photographs in her house, curious about which she'll choose.

"I also want both names on the headstone, Volvinsky and Martin, I think it makes more sense."

Juliette kept her married name after her divorce but had to revert to her maiden name after her retirement. The French authorities had discovered she didn't have her ex-husband's official permission to keep his name after their divorce. And since Dimitri was deceased, she couldn't ask. She was very upset about this, and it bothered me too. Had she remarried, she may have changed her name, or used both, but under that circumstance, it was as if Juliette Volvinsky's identity was stolen, erased, never to be hers again.

Why she wants both names is immediately clear to me. Few people would know who Juliette Martin was. Fortunately, it's legal to have a moniker on a grave in France, so both names are allowed on the headstone. It's a consolation for what had been, at the time, yet another letdown.

As for the memorial photograph, I get it. People walking by her grave would recognize one of two names or remember her face.

From this, I wonder whether we may all fear leaving nothing behind, not even proof of who we were.

"Don't worry… It will be done." I say this looking at Corinne who doesn't comment.

She might find her mother's demand materialistic, but since she says nothing against it, I assume she agrees. Besides, hearing Juliette expressing her last wishes makes me a witness.

As for the *dress-up* matter, Juliette shared a strange dream, a few mornings ago. She was choosing the clothes she'd wear for her burial and decided on the "cream white blazer she bought in the States." I wonder whether her unspoken reticence about the color of the lining has to do with that blazer.

"The other day, you talked about the white blazer you bought in the States. Do you—"

She interrupts again. "My blazer is not white, it's cream white. And cream white won't look good with the plain white of the lining."

What? I get it, but I am the only one smiling.

Her dilemma about the colors wasn't meant as a joke; she would go in her own style.

Corinne approaches her mother and kisses her forehead then must go back to work. I can't leave Juliette alone right now. She'll have enough time to think of today before she falls asleep. It's now just the two of us. I sit very close to her and try to join her in her 'bubble' because only *she* knows how it is in *there*.

I ask how she is feeling. She says she is relieved that things are taken care of. Then I suddenly have the urge to explain my apparent casual demeanor of today.

I've been in such a controlled mode, I behaved as if everything was normal, but I am not taking any of this lightly. I did what had to be done because I didn't want her to worry anymore; besides, it felt so surreal to be at the funeral home, and I struggled through it, as did Corinne. The truth is, I am sad, I am upset… I can't stop talking. Even if it's wrong to bring it all back to how I feel. Her hand on my cheek puts an end to my rambling.

"I know… but there was no other way. It helps so much that you can do this… that there are two of you to make decisions… I don't know what I would have done without you."

"I wish I could do more. I can't get off my mind that…" *how do I say this?* "…nothing will ever be the same when I come to visit my family. I can't imagine that next time you will be… uh… there." *Have I said too much?* I wonder.

"It will still be nice… I know you'll bring me flowers." She pauses. "Remember, it's my destiny… I can't go against it."

It will still be… nice? Her words resonate in a strange way. I can't reconcile my sadness with her gratitude for the flowers I'll bring to her grave. She is beyond the fight, beyond the revolt. She trusts her destiny. And she is repentant. She might not be in the religious state of grace, but I sense the divine in her words, and in her voice too.

I lean over to hug her and say goodbye, careful not to pull on the IV tube. She looks tired. I am not ill like her, but I am tired too.

I can't wait to go back to my parents and sit at the kitchen table. I can't wait to take in the comforting aroma of my mother's steaming vegetable soup made from scratch. I am grateful but feel guilty that I can get away from the hospital whereas Juliette can't.

My parents ask a few questions, but I refrain from volunteering information. Juliette's situation is a reminder, to them and to me, of their mortality.

Lying in bed that evening, I think of the new insights I gained into what Juliette calls *destiny*.

I map it as what happens between birth and death, as our personal bubble of sorts. One that grows with us until it bursts and releases us. It bursts according to our unique place in the universe for some, or God's will for others. Juliette's bubble is about to burst, and mine will someday too, because we are destined to make space for new ones. I imagine these bubbles as invisible, mysterious vessels powered by the unique energy that transports us through life, and to a mysterious destination, an ever-perplexing, incomprehensible universe. Again, it may be to the absolute end of all life for some, to the beginning of a heavenly life for others, or to another dimension for yet others.

I can't say what it is for Juliette, other than after struggling to find it, she seems to be connecting with 'something.'

CHAPTER 26
Pondering Faith

OUR CONVERSATIONS ABOUT death would make me yet again ponder my convoluted relationship with supreme power, with God. Unlike the faith intuitively ingrained in people raised in a religious family, unconditional faith has been a struggle for me. What's natural and unquestionable to them isn't to me because it wasn't part of my upbringing, of my family culture. What's inherently true for 'believers' isn't to me and vice versa. I eventually had to accept that.

I was baptized and attended church with my friends every Sunday until *confirmation* when I was seven years old and *communion solennelle* at twelve, but I wasn't a practicing Christian after that. My worship of the creation of the world is spiritual, but not that of a dogmatic religion. When I pray or thank God, I connect with 'him' more as the evolutive power that created planet Earth and the universe. I am grateful to have faith in that divine supreme power because it's all that I am afforded.

When I had to reconcile the nevertheless pious wellness that I felt when I attended mass with my resistance to dogmatic faith, I realized it was revered fascination more than piousness.

I feel reverence in a church as a sacred place, from my experience in the church of my village. That reverence was born from a solemn ritual; walking down the nave toward the allegorical mural painted high on the curved wall behind the altar, the twinkling candles, the glowing stained-glass windows, the pervading scent of wood wax combined with the resinous hints of incense, the chanting of mysterious Latin words, and after mass, the feeling of fulfillment and wholeness as I walked out, under the church imposing pillars and arches. A grandeur likely intended to generate that reverence.

Elated, I would emerge into daylight at the sound of pealing bells. Yet that elation may have had as much to do with my fervor at singing in the choir as it had with the sense of self that I gained from this space secluded from the life outside the church's walls. I felt joy, serenity, and a sense of belonging too.

Most of my friends' parents didn't attend church either. Yet, most villagers did before the First World War and its atrocities, before an acquired rancor was passed on. Too much was lost and blind faith in God was too much to ask.

As an adult, I eventually accepted to be 'born again,' but resistance returned, and I felt like an impostor. I do not *believe* as I 'should' since there is only *one* way to be a 'true Christian.' Even sought out heartily, total surrender escapes me, doesn't feel right, as did confession that had a young me pick from a list of sins those that sounded serious enough to ask for forgiveness. It would have made more sense to ask for forgiveness over my impertinence at my mother, but it seemed too simple a sin.

Today, whether I feel contrition or gratitude, both stem from the reliance on something bigger than myself. To the 'God' out there.

Even the priest of my youth was an enigma. Yet, his outreach to young souls was limited to the tools he was given.

On the one hand, he was approachable despite the implicit power of his black cassock, and young enough to play ball in the church square when we took breaks from catechism classes, or during *in situ* daily 'retreats.'

On the other hand, he was unapproachable when he discouraged my questions about the enigmatic Virgin Mary, or the miraculous multiplications of the fish and loaves, not to mention the complexity of the Holy Trinity. I wondered why God made it so complicated for children to understand this. Why should I accept what I couldn't understand when no one seemed to know how to explain it? Later, I would of course face how deep is the meaning of *faith*.

As an adolescent, I reconciled myself with the stories of the Bible, only metaphorically. I accepted the parables as I did the fables in the books of my childhood, for the moral values they imparted.

Still struggling and somewhat repentant for my lack of unconditional faith, I eventually found the same solace, reverence, enchantment, and spiritual awe in nature.

The shafts of light through the trees are the candles, the sun dawning and setting glows like stained glass, and the scents of the forest contribute the olfactory element. And although the chirpiness of bird songs can never replace the entrancing monophonic Gregorian chants, I feel the same sense of the divine as I did in the church. I would likely feel the same way in a mosque; I did in a synagogue, and at a Balinese shrine too. And my *namaste* after meditation also takes me *there* when, sitting on my heels, my chin bows to my joined hands before they rise to my forehead, my arms naturally extending into a forward bow until my fingers reach the floor. In grateful reverence to my creator, that of Earth and humanity.

As it stands, the feeling of peace and wholeness from acknowledging the 'natural God in me' is sustaining enough. It wasn't easy to reconcile the church's doctrinal rejection of the evolutionary theory, but I respect those with that belief.

However, that the Bible—hence the New Testament—be a reinterpretation of the Old Testament isn't helping. However, since the Romans used educated guesswork to interpret hieroglyphs, the science of the future might help interpret the 'Word of God' in a more plausible way; one that would unite humanity instead of dividing it.

From this, I believe that human beings were given a divine mission in their earthly life: to honestly seek one's truth. This implies that we are not all born to live religiously equal.

Perhaps a godly power led mankind to create different religions, to test our righteousness in seeking and accepting our unique truth, and to challenge our tolerance toward other people's beliefs.

It shuffled my mind to encounter Christianity as just another creation story in the college mythology course, previously mentioned. Christianity… a religion that imposed itself on others who had their own divine beliefs. As if there should be only lambs in the animal kingdom—the Christian metaphor for mankind. This coercion is how *I* relate to the original sin.

Meanwhile, times are changing in surprising ways. In France, some churches have reverted to Latin, traditionalist worshippers lamenting the modern tongue, and resenting a simplified decorum that 'diminished their fervor,' they say. Solemn rituals generate a mysterious bond that helps connect with our inner self, as contemplation does, but when that ritual disappears so does the bond.

The fact that the Pope approved only twenty parallel congregations adds to the complexity of the traditional Catholic church. Why such diversity to spread the 'Word of God'? Jesus was a simple man, only with great wisdom. The 'church' he referred to was of supreme power, but not of ostentatious wealth. As the fourteenth Dalai Lama does, I believe in the thought that 'true religion means having a good heart.' In that sense, the 'church' is in each one of us; it's the essence of who we are; it's living as righteous a life as we can. It's believing in redemption because stumbling happens even to the fittest of walkers.

In the end, it might be in mankind's ultimate destiny to understand that there is only one creator for all; and that God's children are Mother Earth's children, first.

CHAPTER 27
The Assignment

JULIETTE HAS ONE last task for Corinne and me: bring clothes from her wardrobe so she can decide on her last 'dress-up.' It's now evident that the 'cream white' blazer issue wasn't entirely meant as a witty comment. And as strange as it is to imagine doing this, choosing the last outfit she'll ever wear is what we must do next.

"Do you remember Sophie's photograph in my living room?" Juliette asks.

"Yes, it's on the shelves by the coffee table."

The photograph in a frame decorated with butterflies was my gift, a way to remember her late daughter, and for a reason I'll give later. I took that picture when Sophie visited us in California.

"Do you want me to bring it to you?"

"You read my mind… yes… I want to take it with me." It's the first time Juliette has mentioned Sophie since my arrival.

I meet Corinne at Juliette's house and park in front of the garage as I usually do. It's February, yet no cheerful primroses or pansies, and no winter flowers greet me by the small gate. I had to justify to Juliette why I prefer the discreet violas to the look-at-me-first pansies: the small perennials bloom into a dainty bunch through the summer whereas the large pansies turn scraggly as soon as the spring is over.

Today, the gate squeaks open onto a lifeless garden. Summer annuals I can no longer identify died in the terra-cotta pots by the front door. As if alluding to the gloom that has grown inside the house.

The round flower bed in the front lawn turned into a strange geometry of stooped black stems and drooped, shapeless flowers. They remind me of the French painter Bernard Buffet, of his distinctive way of expressing realism in a technique of thick, elongated black lines in landscapes, portraits, and still lifes. His gloomy art spoke to me in my late teens when depression darkened my mind. His view of fine art had further impressed my uninitiated sensibilities. A painting is not meant to be talked about or analyzed, but to be felt, Buffet once explained. Sadly, he felt and endured his dark lines until they clawed beyond the canvas, to his suicide.

I see that same despair in the black outline of Juliette's lifeless flower bed. *My* white rosebush needs pruning, its naked thorny branches screaming at the sky.

I ring the bell and wait until Corinne opens the door. We briefly hug then I follow her into the living room where she has been sorting the mail on the dining table. The rolling shutters of the French window are up but the traditional wooden shutters are closed. It hits me that this usually bright room now stands in darkness. Corinne accepts to let some daylight in and reminds me that we must watch the time; she must go back to work. While she keeps sorting the mail, I look around.

Photographs on the glass and black metal shelving remind me to take the frame with the butterflies. Before I put it in my handbag, I look at Sophie. Sophie, who had regained control over her drug addiction, then; Sophie, who hadn't relapsed, again. Sophie, who hadn't had twins, yet. Sophie, who was still living. Like her mother's, her wavy dark hair frames her face, her brown eyes endearing as always. The photograph sends me the same half-smile as her mother's sometimes: an enigmatic smile that makes me hold her stare as if I held her destiny in my hand. As if I had the power to take her back in time so that fatal day never happened.

I turn to the dark blue armchair and, for a split second only, Juliette is sitting there, talking. Behind in the corner is the piano. Next to the sofa is the ornate, white wood-and-marble end table that Juliette promised to Sophie—who wouldn't live long enough to make it her own. On it is a silver tray with two dark blue porcelain cups from India, a silver teapot, and a plant. On that table is also my gift of a skinny, white crystalline-marble bear sitting on its bum, that she found 'absolutely irresistible.' On the coffee table matching the shelving, Juliette always had a seasonal plant, or flowers—often from her garden.

Four white cane-back chairs anchor the white square table in the dining room area, and a large mirror replicates the paintings on the opposite wall. Above the credenza, the largest of her paintings encapsulates the realist genre. Bought at a private gathering with the artist, we had commented on the details of a pleasant lifestyle—people riding horses by an elegant country house in a pastoral setting.

Juliette likely chose the still life hanging next to the mirror for the fruit spilling from a dish or about to roll off the table, so much more interesting than piled up in a bowl. Three smaller frames hang in a geometrical pattern, a Russian icon that may have belonged to her mother-in-law, a naïve painting that brings the word *pueblo* to mind, and a collage of family photographs.

She managed to soften the look of the audio equipment in a corner by assembling a CD/DVD tower topped with a sculpted wood tree, likely a memento of a trip, and a floor lamp with a white shade and a tall cylindrical base, made of that transparent material called *Lucite*. Next to those and on a similar stand, a plant balances the energy. Juliette would have simply said: *it looks better this way*.

I would later find the story behind her new audio system.

February 2011

My dear Marie-Claude,

After much consideration, I have finally decided to cancel my trip to Jordan and Syria, considering the situation in Egypt, which is not evolving positively. With the riots that are spreading throughout the entire country, I wouldn't feel at ease in these turbulent regions where one never knows what to expect. It's not the best environment to have a good time. So, I am staying at home. Instead, I bought a new LED television (beautiful), and a Blu-ray DVD player, and a new radio/CD player for my car. And, to top it all, I am getting electric rolling shutters for the living room window. This took a toll on my finances, but I am very pleased with my new acquisitions. I am left with the pleasant prospect of a trip to Peru in September unless there is a revolution there too. I also plan to spend four days in London in May. "Never say die!"

Juliette

She wrote the message in French and ended it with the English expression, *Never say die!* as we often did when English was more expressive than French. I must admit, I thought she meant to write "Never say never" but, she was an editor. Looking it up reminded me that there is no such thing as total bilingualism.

As I revisit what's around me, I linger on familiar objects such as the small, whimsical bronze hippopotamus on the coffee table, whose incongruous beauty I have always been fond of. All are gathered in attractive ensembles, avoiding clutter.

What will happen to what Corinne calls: "stuff, material things that replace spirituality"? The thought reminds me of the words of a flea market dealer: "What older folks don't want to sell cheap now, their children will give away later." As disheartening as it was to hear, his bluntness got my attention.

As I look at my friend's 'treasures' I realize that the valuables we collect and the knick-knacks we accumulate are our stories, not our children's, who have their own stories. Still, it's disconcerting that their generation often prefers mass-produced items, with no stories, and so affordable that they are easily tossed and replaced. Perhaps they are intuitively refusing to burden their lives with our past when their present can be so overwhelming already.

In our home in Vancouver, family pieces that didn't make the cut because of style and space were donated or are in limbo in the basement. Still, I am sensitive to family heirlooms as reminders that we stand on the shoulders of our elders.

Ironically, sooner or later past trends come back, with a designer twist. Vintage objects get a new life, giving substance to the minimalistic style of a modern environment. Fashion brings back styles from our youth, for better or for worse. Even wallpaper is making a comeback, as a warming element to the industrial and deconstructed look.

In Juliette's home, I am not aware of any object that was her mother's or grandmother's. I would later find out why. Instead, Juliette put a personal touch on her contemporary style with meaningful artisanal pieces.

Because they tell a story.

As I stand in her mother's house, Corinne's criticism is still on my mind, waiting like the mail she is still sorting. I feel pressed to defend my friend because this might be my last opportunity to be alone with her daughter. I wonder when to begin that conversation as I watch Corinne open envelopes, glance at the content, and separate it into growing piles. Not wanting to interrupt, I am heading to the kitchen when I come upon a painting; two women sit, one on a sofa and the other in an armchair, perhaps in a cabaret, and both look in the same direction. The painting is familiar since I have one almost identical.

Juliette and I came across a few of these paintings in Spain, at the Marbella Rastro, a flea market, farmers' market, and outlet for cheap resort fashion essentials. Set on the hill between the bullring and a terraced shopping center with cafés and restaurants, it was the place to be seen on Saturday morning, and where even socialites showed off inexpensive, trend-of-the-moment clothing and jewelry, along with their unmistakable designer pieces.

A series of that same painting may have been the work of art school students, each one showing an artist's attempt at rendering the best composition, light, and colors of the same subject. The women's attire and hairstyle, and the Art Deco coffee table, suggest a scene from *Les Années Folles*—the Roaring Twenties—when prosperity swept the Western world in a frenzy for culture, and when women's fashion took an alluring turn. Juliette and I loved the two women's dresses, and their hair, loosely curled for one, and square cut above the neck for the other.

We never decided which woman was her or me, but Juliette would have likely chosen the one with the cascading curls, claiming that a headband across her forehead wouldn't suit her face structure. In my home, the version of that painting is a landmark in the memories of our friendship.

In the kitchen, the white IKEA cabinets, bought for this then-new house, show signs of wear. I recall Juliette's exuberance after sort of smuggling from Switzerland one or two components at a time. Her country-French-style kitchen isn't meant as a showcase, although today's French designs are more linear and minimalistic, and more adapted to smaller spaces. Above all, her kitchen is convivial, inviting you to sit down for a chat while the tea is steeping.

The toaster stays in a corner of the counter, next to the percolator, because she uses both for breakfast. An earthenware bowl holds kitchen utensils, easily reachable from her gas stove. A kettle stands on one of the four burners, next to the pressure cooker, often used for her signature *blanquette de veau*—a veal stew with a cream sauce that she served over tagliatelle pasta.

Among the cookbooks on a wall-mounted shelf, next to the fridge, are Indian ones, likely gifts from Mallick. He gave her such gifts when they lived together and even after they no longer did, a hint at their complicated relationship.

Small kitchen gadgets bought on trips were also the kind of gifts she gave to friends: my timer from New York, in the shape of a red apple; a flamboyant apron, from New Orleans; not that I could forget a cookbook from Québec with eighty recipes just for chicken.

Above the small table set perpendicularly to the wall hangs a painting of Provencal dancers, by her neighbor Daria. Lace curtains with a bucolic theme give partial privacy from the single-lane road through her small neighborhood. The hedge along her property is low enough so she can wave at neighbors walking by when she stands at the sink. She has a friendly relationship with her neighbors—although I know of one story to the contrary.

It may have been three years before she fell ill that Juliette disagreed with Daria's husband because of the quaint wooden shed he built on *his* property, yet away from their double fence. Juliette complained that it clashed with… something, the adjacent pasture, or the neighborhood, I forget which. One day, after she insisted that I see what she meant, even on tiptoes I couldn't see over her hedge. She then admitted she could only see the shed through a gap in the foliage. She never talked about it again and I wonder from what nook or cranny in her mind such a futile fuss came.

Corinne joins me in the kitchen and opens the fridge. Having occasionally overnighted in the house, she checks the expiration dates on yogurts. This reminds me of last November when I took Juliette grocery shopping, and of the soy yogurts she couldn't find. Corinne leaves a bag of perishables by the front door, and I follow her back into the living room. I feel pressed for time since we must still select clothes. I take a last look at my friend's favorite room before it returns to darkness.

"Look at this! All this…. *stuff*." Corinne uses that word again, sweeping the air with her arm. She has no idea she just prompted me to speak up and let her know that I find her judgment of her mother unfair.

CHAPTER 28
A Cathartic Talk

I FACE CORINNE, hesitating. Will the discussion we are about to have be too upsetting for her? I wonder. Why did she revert to the negativity of her relationship with her mother, her emails suggesting otherwise? In the end, not only does my loyalty to Juliette guide me, but I feel that Corinne needs to sort out their mutual resentment. But will she be receptive to my comments? It's my only opportunity to find out.

"Corinne…" My grave tone of voice gets her attention. "We need to talk about what you just said… again… about your mother."

She looks at me, tiredness furrowing her brows. I empathize, but I must keep talking.

"I know your mother's fears, her feelings, and her regrets… and I find your judgment of her very unfair. So… unless you know what I know, you won't be able to let her go in peace… and you might not find peace either."

To my relief, Corinne looks surprised but willing to hear more.

I say her name again, with bold yet compassionate determination. "Your mother's life isn't empty, as you said, but it's lonely. She suffers from solitude, loneliness, aloneness…

whatever you want to call it. But what you call *stuff*—" I make air quotes "—are not meaningless things. They make up her cocoon… woven over a lifetime… and always available for emotional comfort when she needs it." I then pause.

What will happen next? Will Corinne get angry and tell me to mind my own business? Instead, calmer than I am, she questions the loneliness I mentioned. When I explain that Juliette would have liked to see her grandchildren regularly, for example, Corinne insists that she did.

"Your mother resented you for rarely allowing a sleepover. Why couldn't you let them spend more time with her?" I know the past can't be undone but I hope she sees my point.

"Pfff… all my mother did with my daughter was show her make-up and clothes and things like that." Corinne's matter-of-fact response again reminds me of her mother.

"Corinne! Your mother is intelligent and cultured and would have done more, but it's hard to do when there is no continuity. She was so happy when you allowed her to take each kid on a trip to Paris."

I am expecting much of Corinne on a day that is already difficult. Frustrated, I didn't sugarcoat my accusations. I pause again, watching her close the wooden shutters in silence until she turns around.

"Yes… I should have let her spend more time with them. I didn't realize she was so lonely… she always talked about—" I hear the spike of annoyance "—all her friends."

"Yes. She has friends. But aging without the closeness of a family weakens a person's confidence. She craved reassurance, the acceptance of a caring family. I'm sorry to be so blunt, but this has been bothering me since we went to the funeral home. I had to talk to you before I leave." I spoke quickly, afraid she or something might interrupt.

I let Corinne ponder my words as she stands still by her mother's dining room credenza, where framed photographs and objects reflect a woman who connected with her space. Then she looks at me, grave and attentive.

"It's important for me to hear this. I need to sort out what has been going on… our differences… you know?" I nod, her words encouraging me to continue.

"There is something else I need to tell you."

This time, Corinne's eyebrows rise.

"You said Sophie felt belittled when your mother visited her in the States." The thought flushes me with both anger and weariness, so I take a deep breath, for I have much to say, again.

Her mother had agonized over Sophie's drug addiction and tried to help her. I ask that she imagines herself in her mother's situation. Living far away, the only times her mother could try to reason with her drug-addicted daughter were during her visits. Confronting Sophie about her lifestyle and pleading with her to get help was all her mother could do under the circumstances. But Sophie couldn't do that, and Juliette may have felt as defeated as Sophie felt belittled. Silence follows my monologue as I remember Sophie, a beautiful young woman trapped by addiction.

I can't resist sharing what's still on my mind.

"Think about it! In San Francisco, your mother bought the same necessities she already bought for Sophie when she lived in San Jose… because Sophie sold them to buy drugs, yet she understood that's what drug addicts do. She was devastated when money was missing from her wallet during her visits.

Because that too is what addiction did to her daughter."

Corinne heaves a deep breath, either from impatience or to say something. I raise my hand to signal I have more to say.

"When Sophie was in rehab in Paris, then doing better until she plunged again, your mother feared every day the phone call that would give her the dreaded news. Then Sophie got better and moved to the States. Things seemed okay until she was pregnant." I pause, remembering vividly Juliette's telephone call in the middle of the night.

"When your mother told me Sophie was expecting twins, she sounded numb, but I imagine her distress when she first heard about it."

I pause again, and Corinne listens with no clear intention of shutting me up.

"What would you have done... visit your drug-addicted daughter and approve of her life? Your mother supported Sophie's decision to move to California... but when things went wrong again, she couldn't act as if she didn't care... as if she only came to California to visit me."

Then I stop talking.

We both look at the floor. I hear her inhaling deeply through her nose and exhaling slowly through her mouth, a learned cleansing breath from her yoga practice. She is letting go of the anger I channeled to her.

My heart is pounding, and I am shaking inside. What happens now? Who will talk first? I am relieved when she does.

"I appreciate your friendship. I don't have anyone with whom to talk about my mother." Her comment surprises me, and it crosses my mind to say it's because she kept her mother at a distance, especially from her friends. But I don't say that.

Moved by her honesty, I let her ponder her words.

Had Corinne had someone to confide in, it may have helped her gain perspective on her rejection of her mother. And although she can't make up for those lost times, I sense a shift in her mind.

"I'm sorry there has been so much anger and miscommunication between us… but my mother hasn't been… easy… you know?"

"I know."

Juliette could be difficult and did have the frustrating habit of taking over a conversation. If she got the slightest bit of attention, she craved more and held on to it harder. She also liked to be right, a sure way to create conflict. Beyond this, there was more to her mother than Corinne knew.

Still, I ask her to understand the hardships that made her mother who she is. She couldn't change her past and it impacted her present. I then want Corinne to imagine her mother through the pain I observed, with one example that will hopefully make her see the point I am trying to make.

On one recent Mother's Day, Corinne invited her mother-in-law but not her mother. As a mother herself, could she understand Juliette's bitterness over this? She made her mother feel as belittled as she said her mother made Sophie feel. After that day, Juliette felt that she didn't matter, not even to her now-only daughter.

"Corinne… I care about your mother, but I also care about you… You are an extension of my friend." I want her to feel my compassion.

The gravity on her face softens; she gets it.

"My friend will be gone soon, but you are here… I hope to

see you when I visit my family. I am sorry I was so tough, but I had to help you understand your mother… so you won't have regrets. It's not too late to acknowledge what went wrong between the two of you. What *you* initiated has already brought you closer. You both need to be at peace when your mother leaves."

I am done speaking.

I look at my watch, aware that it's time to move on. Should I give her space and offer to meet her outside or back at the hospital? Yet we still have a mission, here.

"Thank you… for being so direct… and truthful. Let's look at her clothes!" Her brave reaction is the answer to my silent question.

CHAPTER 29

The Ultimate Dress-Up

THE SOUND OF our steps on the wooden staircase to the upper floor reminds me that they became an obstacle to Juliette. She had to crawl up or step down backward because she was determined to sleep in her bedroom. A bed taking over her living room would have been the ultimate sign of defeat, emotionally if not creatively.

The first thing I see on the landing is my favorite of Sophie's paintings, a talent she likely inherited from her father.

It's a scene from Geneva Old Town with a simplified version of Cathédrale Saint Pierre in the background. Yellow, red, and ocher illuminate the foliage of trees, suggesting that it's autumn. But the heart of the painting is Sophie's interpretation of the merry-go-round, where I used to take our children when we lived in Geneva. The rich décor of the carousel matches the bright colors of the trees. I liked it so much I commissioned Juliette's son to paint one for me.

Thoughtful, he added two women—meant to be Juliette and me. They were looking not at children merrily riding around—there were none in the painting—but at one white horse, a seal nosing a ball, an elephant, and an octopus. Until I wrote about it, I didn't notice this singularity, having been mostly attracted by the overall colorful composition of the theme. I also noticed the date: 2004, ten years before his mother would die.

The cheerful painting often brings back nostalgic memories, though. I hear in my head the band organ music, the same as that of the circus or the *fêtes foraines*—the traveling funfairs—that came to our village. Today, mind-blowing rides provide an adrenaline rush that resets the mind, as per the exhilarating reactions of those riders. As if the psyche craved that fight-or-flight reaction, now a natural high from that induced fear.

Back to Juliette's house.

On the upper level of her duplex are two bedrooms, a functional room—with a daybed, an ironing board, and other conveniences—and a bathroom. A multipurpose room runs the depth of the house and was Mallick's space, and where Juliette still has a desk.

Memorabilia on shelves mingle with books and other framed photographs. Paintings and sketches animate the walls. Some are by Sophie or her brother, and a few sketches are by Juliette herself. After retiring, she took drawing classes and framed and hung a few of her sketches in an attractive display.

In her bedroom, the intricate silk bedspread—one of Mallick's gifts—attests to the Indian tradition of recycling sumptuous vintage wedding saris into bedspreads, murals, and cushions. Unmatched in style, a small chest of drawers and a vanity table display sentimental items: small boxes, jewelry, and framed photographs of her younger years, creating warmth and meaning to her surroundings.

Corinne opens the wall-to-wall closet and I immediately freeze. I can't focus on any of the clothes, knowing what they are for. I also wonder what questions our choices will trigger in

Juliette's mind—why this garment and not another?

Many people had to do this, but it's my first time, and no one is dead yet.

Then none of the dresses we pull out seem appropriate. A black cocktail dress appears too festive, and a casual one lacks a ceremonial vibe. Long dresses weren't Juliette's style; still, I am drawn to long-sleeve blouses and pants, for the tranquilizing thought that they'd protect her body.

We finally select a Chinese blouse with braided loops secured by knot buttons across the chest. Juliette's enthusiasm for her trip to China is evident in her unusual choice of its apple-green color. We pair it with black wide-leg crepe pants, and we don't forget the cream white blazer.

As we keep looking, I wonder whether Juliette would want to look *comme il faut*—it means *following the rules*, but with a hint of derision—or a more free-spirited style. I catch myself thinking that she must look appropriate as if she must abide by some social etiquette.

Corinne is considering a light gray wool sweater from Peru that I pair with a pink shawl for its softening color. Unsure of what else to take, we add other pants, a couple of blouses, and her favorite black tops.

Next, we hesitate on the shoes after passing on high heels and ankle boots. I am pleased to find a pair of pink ballerina-style flats with clusters of gold dust, but Corinne looks at them with shocked amazement until she points to the design. The clusters of gold dust represent skulls.

I am not surprised that Juliette found a way to follow this trend—borrowed from Gothic fashion, an ancient Germanic subculture. The dystopian hint doesn't escape me, and Juliette would have gloated over this. The unexpected encounter briefly lightens our mood.

From the clothes laid on her bed, I imagine Juliette's indecision over which to choose, and combining them in her unique way. Then Corinne points to a maroon silk blazer that doesn't fit her, and that Juliette wants me to have, something I was not aware of.

Juliette had it tailored in China, her last trip. She likely took time to compare the silk fabrics before settling on yet another nuanced color: maroon. I can't help thinking that the tailor took her measurements when cancer had already taken hold of her body. She never got to wear this blazer, nor receive the compliment that would have spawned yet another story.

What time is it? I don't remember hearing the small gate moan on its hinges or Corinne locking the front door and getting into her car. I don't remember driving by the neighborhood mailboxes where Juliette and I began our goodbye, last November.

Back at the hospital, the moment we enter Juliette's room is as awkward as when we returned from the funeral home. Corinne holds the garment bag, hesitating about what to do until Juliette points to the patient cabinet by the window. She then leaves to go back to work.

I place Sophie's framed photograph on the nightstand. Juliette says she thought of taking a photo of her whole family with her, along with Sophie's, but she changed her mind.

"It didn't feel right… to take them with me… in death."

Later, this would remind me of my high school literature course and of Montaigne—the French Renaissance philosopher—who devised life and death and conceived the thought that *we trouble our life with thoughts about death and our death with thoughts about life*.

CHAPTER 30
Remembering Sophie

THE NEXT DAY, Juliette mentions Sophie when she sees me glance at the framed photograph on her nightstand. I even detect acceptance in her voice, as if approaching death allows her to make peace with that painful memory. As if she can finally face her youngest daughter's fate.

In the past, Juliette rarely mentioned Sophie, and only once did she comment on how she took her life. It's the kind of tragedy that one must learn to live with, for it never leaves.

Had she started that conversation during one of my visits, it would have been difficult to move on. She didn't want our time together to be overtaken by sadness and, for my part, I avoided conversations that might revive her grief.

I would get a different perspective on such a loss from a neighbour-friend. When we reunited years after we all moved away, Angie noticed my hesitation as I recalled our children playing together. "It's okay to talk about Matthew," she said. "It's comforting to have him in our memories." Those may not have been her exact words, but it was her message.

Angie learned not to fear the motorcycle accident that killed her son. But Juliette couldn't face the ghastly side of her youngest daughter's suicide. She never talked about it, the specter of guilt constantly hovering. Angie's soul-searching helped her tame her pain and cherish the memory of her son. She shares her loss with her child's father. As the sole parent Juliette's loss was all hers.

Today, Juliette seems appeased. I wonder whether it's due to our long conversation yesterday, to the soothing thought of reuniting with her daughter's spiritual energy. After all, she did say, "It would be comforting to believe in something."

Juliette had waited until her youngest daughter turned fifteen to divorce, as she said she would the day we met. Her youngest child would be old enough to care for herself while living with her older brother and sister, and their father. Still, Juliette was upset about this practical arrangement caused by Dimitri's refusal to move out, and the cost of a legal battle. Her rationale was that it would keep the children in the family home.

Unfortunately, *practical* didn't mean *simple*. Corinne would remind me that her mother left without notice; no one knew where she was for a while. I had forgotten that Juliette was in hiding when I visited her at her friend's place. She had run away after another explosive fight with Dimitri. Leaving was her way to protect her children; hiding was to protect herself.

Juliette's plan backfired, though, unfolding as she feared rather than hoped. With no parental stability, the children turned to their friends, some perhaps in broken homes too.

Sophie got into drugs, went into rehab in Paris, then moved to California. There, she reunited with her half-brother (from Dimitri's first ex-wife). There, she also met a handsome man a few years older. I met him after driving Sophie back to San Jose, following her first visit to our home in California. I thought he was sensible and attentive, and I was happy to give Juliette encouraging news. Sophie had found a new life.

Sophie was a sensitive young woman with fine features and a gentle voice. She wasn't tall like her sister nor thin like her mother but of an attractive middle size. She was studying art on and off, so after her move to California, I invited her to a lunch combined with an art show by local artists, in the country-club community where we lived.

After she settled in the guest room, she asked about the roses on the desk table and was surprised they were from my garden and for her to enjoy. We chatted while she drank cup after cup of coffee with cream and loads of sugar. She looked fragile but well and apparently clean of drugs.

Like her father, Sophie was an artist. She painted or used crayons in her expressive style. I had hoped she would sell a few pieces that day, but after selling 'only two,' she felt rejected. It was beyond her understanding that the apparently well-off women didn't buy more from the artists. I explained that people look at art more than they buy it, even if they like it.

Back at the house, and inspired by her portfolio, I commissioned several watercolors, depicting the activities enjoyed in our family: American football, tennis, music, golf, and horse vaulting. She drew them in an eye-catching conceptual way. But the piece that captivated me in her portfolio was a drawing of an old woman sitting at a water's edge.

Sophie used chalk to draw it in three colors, the medium-brown paper acting as a fourth, binding the woman to the void around her. That brown undertone deepens the azure blue of the woman's long skirt as well as the pink patches peeking from its pleats. White chalk illuminates her blouse and headscarf, the ribbons of clouds uncurling in the medium-brown sky, and the crests of waves purling the shore of the medium-brown waters; that white subliminally enlivening the dimmed scene like glimmers of hope.

I noticed her technique of letting the medium-brown paper do the work. Sophie had outlined the woman's face and arms with a graphite pencil, but inside these lines, the paper contributes its medium-brown shade to represent a woman of color.

I was drawn to the overall contrast between the vibrancy and gloom of her work.

The bohemian skirt, the roomy blouse with puff sleeves, and the headscarf tied at the nape of the woman's neck evoke different ethnicities, perhaps that of a Russian peasant in mishappen shoes, oversized like wooden clogs. She sits crouched on a log or a boulder on a shore, perhaps that of an ocean. Her elbows rest on her knees splayed under her skirt, her forearms stretched forward, and her hands joined beyond. She is in profile, looking down and appearing lost in her thoughts, perhaps dreaming of what lies beyond the unreachable horizon.

I wanted to know this woman. Know why she exudes such lassitude and hopelessness.

Sophie had conceived this black woman in Paris when she was in a 'dark place,' she said. The subliminal analogy doesn't escape me that lost souls know no colorism.

I knew Sophie referred to her drug addiction. I told her this sketched woman was the auspicious symbol of a troubled past that was no longer hers.

She, Sophie, had crossed that water and reached the shore of a new life, pushed, or pulled beyond the horizon. If that woman reflected Sophie—feeling hopeless and wishing she could be on that faraway shore—she, Sophie, had made the journey. She was no longer that woman.

But I couldn't have imagined that she didn't make that journey alone, that the hurdles in her past would be the same as those in her future. Neither could I have imagined that she would cut short the obstacle course of her drug addiction.

Today, her art piece hangs in our powder room. As odd as that choice might be, guests see it in a quiet place, where only one person goes at a time, in the same crouched position as the old woman. It might bring a smile to some, and deeper thoughts to others.

Sometimes, I look at it with sadness for the precious life that was lost. Other times, it's with relief; Sophie is free of the demons that hounded her. Drug addiction had held like the talons of an eagle do; it didn't let go until it was all over.

After that summer luncheon, Sophie celebrated part of Thanksgiving Day with us, amused that she'd have two turkey dinners in one day; with us and with her half-brother, who'd moved to Oakland—thirty minutes away and the city connected to San Francisco by the Bay Bridge.

After six months in San Jose, Sophie and her boyfriend then moved to San Francisco. We occasionally talked on the phone and met for lunch in the city. She attended an art school, earning money posing nude for other drawing art classes. Remaining still for long periods was challenging but the effort was worth her newly toned body, as she saw it.

Juliette visited a few months later and immediately saw evidence of Sophie's drug use. What she owned in San Jose was gone—sold or traded. Crushed but resigned, Juliette helped her daughter recreate a home, so she would be safe, warm, and fed for a while. But their time together wasn't without contradictions.

On the one hand, Sophie was comforted by her mother's presence. On the other hand, she stole from her again. Juliette was aware of her addicted daughter's constant obsession with finding ways to buy drugs. Before Sophie went to rehab in Paris, even Mallick's cashmere winter coat had disappeared. I don't know whether Sophie had confessed, or whether Juliette had used her perceptiveness, but I vaguely recall Mallick hoping to buy it back from a second-hand store in Geneva.

Two years later, Juliette's phone call woke me in the middle of the night. She forgot about the nine-hour time difference between France and California.

"Sophie is pregnant," she blurted out.

"What? No…!"

"Her boyfriend is the father."

That detail sounded somewhat odd, but stunned by the news, I tried to find something positive to say. Sophie's pregnancy would help her get a grip on her life.

"She's expecting twins." Her calm was shocking.

Sitting on my bed, I pulled my comforter over my head as I tried to wrap my mind around this double pregnancy. Juliette expected my reaction and stayed silent. She already went through the shock, including worrying about babies born from an addict mother, plus the ensuing financial implications. Sophie's boyfriend had been married before and Juliette suspected he'd moved to California due to some financial trouble. Clearly, she would be the main provider.

I was so stricken that I cursed.

As always, Juliette focused on the positive. Sophie was born in the United States—a fact I had forgotten—the expectant mother and then her babies were eligible for social services.

But a series of complications were to arise.

A few months after the birth of the twin girls, their father left, moving back to Michigan, for a reason unclear to me. It devastated Juliette who worried about the babies' safety. Yet, from their phone conversations, Sophie seemed to have regained control.

When Juliette met her granddaughters, she was slapped with evidence to the contrary—pills and alcohol under Sophie's mattress. Juliette's only consolation was that Child Protective Services would have taken the little girls away had Sophie neglected them.

Once more, Juliette provided what her daughter and granddaughters needed. And although she wished better for the babies than the playpen they were sleeping in, social services likely judged it practical and safe.

A few days into Juliette's visit, Sophie stole from her mother again—not all the money in her wallet, it would have been too noticeable, but also toiletries, clothing, and a book.

Shortly after Juliette's return to France, Sophie sold everything and joined her daughters' father, at his parents' Michigan home.

For the first time, Juliette had hope.

Her granddaughters lived surrounded by family. Juliette even had the support of a clan—invited to stay at the family home on her first visit there. The children's father had a job, and the situation was on an acceptable course until the couple separated again. It was Juliette's turn to provide Sophie and her daughters with a place to live. Life wasn't easy, but it went on until one day, all hell broke loose. Sophie committed suicide.

At the time, Juliette and I hadn't been in contact for a while. There was some frustration in our relationship, mainly on my part. I too needed a good listener, but didn't feel heard, yet her life with Mallick was somewhat stable then. I deeply regretted my attitude.

As a result of our lack of communication, I received the devastating news in the mail, one month later. It was by way of Sophie's memorial program, with a poem about the short life of a butterfly—hence my gift of the photo frame. In total disbelief, I immediately called Juliette.

One of her then eight-year-old twin granddaughters found their mother hanged in the attic. Juliette received the news she'd feared since her daughter was a teenage drug addict.

I was horrified and devastated by all it meant for my friend. All I could do was write.

Vancouver, October 2003

Dear Juliette and family,

It is with great sadness that we think of Sophie today,

But it is with fondness that we will remember her,

Thanks to some of the times we spent together.

When we moved from California to Canada, her artwork followed us,

such as her whimsical sketches representing sports and hobbies.

Sophie was so gifted.

She was also very sensitive.

On her first visit, she was touched by the fresh flowers in her bedroom.

She liked the hill behind our house.

It reminded her of "The Little House on the Prairie."

I used to tease her about how white and sweet she liked what she called coffee!

On one Thanksgiving, she had an early dinner with us and was amused that she'd have another later one with [her half-brother].

On another occasion, I drove her back to [San Jose].

[Her then-boyfriend] *met us for dinner on the pier.*

They were so caring for each other.

And then, 'once upon a time' two beautiful little girls were born.

They, too, will be sensitive to lovely things and have talents of their own.

But the final separation is difficult…

Always remember that Sophie is now forever a free and caring spirit… watching over her loved ones.

With much love to you all,

Marie-Claude & Jim and the whole family

Juliette then coordinated help with the children's father and grandparents. Then complications and worries kept finding her.

First, the grandfather died and a few months later the grandmother's decision had the consequences of a tsunami. After what must have been a serious disagreement with her children, she sold the family home and relocated across the country, to Las Vegas.

Juliette's only contact was now her granddaughters' father.

She already resented his entitlement during his visits to France with the girls and found his attitude about money increasingly upsetting. Even when the twins were old enough to travel as unaccompanied minors, he wouldn't allow it unless Juliette paid for his airline ticket. As it turned out, a few months after she died, he came to France with his daughters. I hope I am wrong to cringe at the thought that he manages their inheritance.

As I remember Sophie, I realize that Juliette may never have openly let herself grieve. If she was depressed, I never saw it, but we didn't see each other regularly. Besides, she avoided the subject.

When we talked, face-to-face or over the telephone, she had that same matter-of-fact tone, guarding her broken heart as if she was afraid to lose some of the pieces.

I thought of this when I read *The Heroine's Journey*. Maureen Murdock draws from Greek mythology to emphasize the importance of letting the pain work through you for as long as it takes, saying: "Only then will deep healing occur."

Like Demeter—the Greek deity who lost her daughter Persephone to Hades, the ruler of the underworld—Juliette must have been inconsolable, but as far as I know, she resisted the healing descent into that darkness.

"One can be upset or frightened by any truth or untruth," Byron Katie says in *A Mind at Home with Itself*. Her advice to tame the pain is to take it back to what it really is or isn't.

If Juliette's simmering anger is an indication, she never tamed that pain. This may also explain her rejection of any form of spirituality; her continual hardships allow no connection to abstract concepts.

I have often wondered whether I was supportive enough, yet our time together made her happy. Still, it saddens me that it may have been my mistake to go along with avoiding talking about Sophie.

CHAPTER 31

Another Pause for Thoughts

CORINNE'S RESENTMENT OF her mother reminds me of the popularized version of Carl Gustav Jung's thought: *what we don't like in others is in us too*. In translation, what the Swiss psychiatrist and psychoanalyst originally wrote in German was: "Everything that irritates us about others can lead us to an understanding of ourselves." The question is: *why does it irritate us?*

It irritates us because *it* unconsciously—from the German *Unbewusste*—triggers a frustrating insecurity in our psyche, a defense mechanism. That emotional reaction is like pushing someone's button by saying or doing what we know (or don't know) will be upsetting. According to Jung, this irritation is a reminder, and evidence, of an inner conflict.

Furthermore, Jung explains that to understand the cause of that irritation we must compare our *self* to… our selfhood, which we cannot do objectively. Either Corinne projected her unconscious feelings of rejection from her mother, or she repressed and rejected what she knew to be true about herself. In any case, sharing with Corinne my perspective of her relationship with her mother somehow helped her make that comparison.

Corinne realized that what makes her cringe about her mother is also in her. Along the same line of thought, in *A New Earth*, Eckhart Tolle hammers the nail even further, by explaining that we might eventually understand this: we do to others what we think others are doing to us. Ouch. Revisiting this broadened and deepened my understanding of my relationships.

I would later share with Corinne what I learned from two years of psychoanalysis, hoping to encourage her to do that work of introspection. It's hard work, hindered by the fear of confronting one's unwavering truth. It usually begins with refusing that a problem exists, it continues with identifying then accepting it, and it hopefully ends with wanting a change. Deepak Chopra says that becoming aware of a problem gives us hope, which allows us to shift our attention from the problem to the solution.

Juliette's state of mind was distorted by her resentment, which she vented as anger. I never witnessed her lashing out at Corinne, but I imagined it from the way she recounted their quarrels, and those with her mother too. Their resentment was one and the same.

Unbeknownst to them, they mirrored each other's unresolved inner conflicts and bitterness, because they never addressed their cause. Juliette's mother unloaded her bitterness on her daughter because her generation coped alone with the memories of an unhappy childhood which, at the time, was usually dominated by a male family member.

Juliette's unresolved conflicts with her mother made her feel unworthy of receiving anything but that resentment. Her persona—the guarded smile for one—was her way to hide that unworthiness, but from that continual state of dissension, something often had to give.

When unresolved conflicts fester within, who we are is not clear even to ourselves. We feel misunderstood. This mental distortion causes a domino effect, from feelings of inadequacy to mental isolation and then to loneliness. I would later discover that what was going on with Juliette was going on with me, too.

I didn't elaborate with Corinne that her mother's inflexibility and defensiveness were the deceiving shields that hid her inner struggles. At the time, I didn't understand it clearly either.

Juliette's parents had broken her trust—the breach of filial love. Her husband turned violent—the loss of romantic love. Her lover of more than two decades never married her—the failure to be loved enough. Her youngest daughter committed suicide—the abnegation of all love of herself.

Juliette's character and mine reflect different influences, but we somehow have similar susceptibilities. Our unconscious minds recognized a kinship, which would later reveal why Juliette and I remained friends for so long despite the distance.

At the time, sharing these complexities with Corinne didn't feel right. And yet, Juliette likely had a reason to share more about herself before she died. Still, I had to process how it related to me before I could pass it on.

CHAPTER 32

Romance in Croatia

OUR CONVERSATIONS OCCASIONALLY bring back memories of Juliette's travels. One day, she mentions Marino. Recounting bits of her romantic adventure in Croatia was a welcome diversion, but the whole story had a deeper meaning.

By then, Juliette and Mallick's relationship had ended. As they both aged, Juliette had reasons to initiate that ending. It wasn't easy, Mallick finding reasons to keep visiting her.

Most of the time, it was to bring the *Herald Tribune*, which irritated Juliette who didn't read newspapers, preferring to watch the news on television. Other times, he pretended to have the latest news from the organization whereas they both received the same monthly newsletter. He also continued to give her things that she 'wanted,' even if he stretched the facts.

That's how, much to her consternation one day, she opened the door to the delivery of a black-lacquered upright piano. I imagine them arguing over the 'surprise,' especially when neither one was totally right nor wrong. Once in passing, Juliette said she wished she had learned music.

They seemed to enjoy such arguments, and I am not sure who enjoyed them the most. Meanwhile, only her grandchildren might have tapped the keys in passing, yet after her diagnosis

Juliette had the piano delivered to Corinne—to ensure it'd stay in the family.

The trip to Croatia happened shortly after Juliette's 'final' breakup with Mallick. After her retirement, she was eager to travel, which they seldom did during their relationship. She also longed to meet new people, to belong to a tribe even if it was a transient diaspora of tourists.

Travel was also the opportunity to find a companion who would be free, so she wouldn't age alone. It was her way to keep Mallick at a distance and make him accept her new freedom.

But as she was to experience, travel to exotic destinations took the mind on an equally exotic journey that yielded only meaningless flings. Some people seek a fantasy romance only to leave problems behind, for the time of a cruise or an overland trip. Juliette didn't want a short-lived relationship; her heart was set on commitment.

And so, on that trip to Croatia perhaps six years before she became ill, Juliette fell head over heels for Marino, the Croatian tour guide. They had instant chemistry, she said.

After Juliette returned home from that first trip to Croatia, they talked every day over the telephone. Marino was planning a business trip to Evian, a spa resort in Haute-Savoie—where the famous Evian water has its spring. He wanted to start a travel agency in Croatia and had contacts there to discuss funding or a partnership of sorts.

I couldn't help suspecting a dash of opportunism in his plan. What a coincidence that it should happen in a provincial town conveniently located less than two hours from Juliette's home. But Juliette was so hopeful that I decided to put my suspicion aside.

After Marino postponed three trips, I advised Juliette to tread carefully in this new relationship. Croatia's tourism was booming, and a whole generation deprived by years of war was dreaming of entrepreneurship.

Juliette, though, didn't doubt Marino's honesty. My friend was enjoying a *joie de vivre* revival and since I didn't know the man, I didn't have the heart to spoil it.

When the Evian deal didn't materialize, and Marino couldn't afford the trip to France, Juliette went back to Croatia. She didn't know for how long, but there was "no reason to stay home when he wanted to see her again," as she justified it. Did she see an opportunity for a steady relationship? After all, he wasn't "some guy met in a bar," as she pointed out. Juliette didn't enjoy bars anyway, so my hunch was that she wanted my approval. I was concerned, but she didn't need my permission.

She briefly rented an apartment until she moved in with him, and then enjoyed their life together—cooking for someone again, exploring the area, and meeting new people. Two months later, Marino introduced her to his mother and even to his daughter, despite his initial reluctance. Juliette felt accepted, nurtured even. Marino's moves impressed me since he was younger than Juliette—a reversal of the situation with Mallick.

One day, she announced she was moving to Croatia. I gasped. I told her to slow down, and not sell her house or she might lose everything if the Marino scenario didn't have a happy ending. Fortunately, she hadn't lost all caution when trusting someone.

During Juliette's three-month stay, I didn't hear much from her until she had to return to France before her tourist visa expired. As days turned into weeks, she had yet to reach Marino by telephone. I don't recall whether they ever talked again, but she eventually wrote to concede the end of their romance.

Juliette was always aware of the obstacles of such a relationship, but she never regretted this short chapter in her life. She was in a free relationship, enjoyed the cultural enrichment of living abroad again, and learned yet another language.

Meanwhile, Mallick had no idea of Juliette's whereabouts. He knew she would be traveling, but not when, where, for how long, and most important to him, whether she would travel alone. The pile of *newspapers* by her front door and her full voicemail box were evidence of his obsessive devotion during her absence.

By keeping Mallick in the dark for three months, Juliette proved she meant what she said. She wanted her freedom. She had reached a time in her life when she wanted to seize the day. And she had done just that.

CHAPTER 33
When Juliette Investigates

JULIETTE TOOK ONE overseas trip every year and traveled in Europe too. She showed me photographs when we got together during my visits to France, plus she always had one exceptional story to tell, although she had three about Peru.

The tour had arrived in Machu Picchu by train, from Cusco, but her visit to the protected UNESCO World Heritage Site was cut short.

With no time to adapt, first to Cusco's high altitude and then to Machu Picchu's lower one, she got sick. She didn't even get off the bus that took her group to the entrance of the famous ruins. Instead, it took her right back to the village of Agua Calientes—overcrowded and renamed Machu Picchu Pueblo. "Obviously a better name for business," she said.

There, nothing went right, even after she felt somewhat better.

Several bridges over a deep gorge got her lost. The jumble of shops and restaurants offered no authenticity. She couldn't find the museum that someone praised—the Museo de Sitio Manuel Chavez Ballon isn't in the pueblo but at Machu Picchu, a thirty-minute walk, or so. And since she didn't know what else to do, she bought a few 'outrageously expensive' souvenirs from zealous shopkeepers. She then gasped at the sight of the Boulangerie de Paris and refused to go in. Under similar circumstances, it would have been my saving grace.

Had she not felt sick, Juliette might have put things in perspective. Among shop owners are former subsistence-living farmers who can now sell their goods to visitors and better care for their families, the more entrepreneurial among them indeed importing mass-produced items.

Until then, Juliette had enjoyed Peru, but the icon of the Inca civilization failed to leave her with the awe-inspiring memory she anticipated.

That trip, however, brought an encounter of a different type. She caught the eye of a fellow traveler.

At first, she had reservations about the handsome man who was traveling alone, but his flirtatious approach, knowledge of history, and music appreciation won her over. Not to mention the fit body of someone who worked "in the law enforcement field" as he described his occupation. I forgot his name unless she never mentioned it. The man didn't wait until the end of the trip to say he wanted to see her after their return to France. They exchanged telephone numbers, and he even promised to call first.

Upon her return, two weeks went by when a frustrated Juliette decided *she* would call him.

Although her calls to his 'direct line' failed, she still wanted to believe she'd made a mistake jotting down the number, and not that he'd given her a bogus one. Either way, she would track him down; after all, unbeknownst to him, Mallick had trained her well to get to the bottom of her suspicions.

Like a female version of Inspector Jacques Clouseau—in

The Pink Panther—she found his name after searching the Internet, although under a different phone number. Furious, she readied herself to confront him, and little did the French Don Juan know whom he'd be dealing with.

She admitted that her hands were shaking, and her heart was pounding when she dialed the number, but she immediately regained control at the sound of the man's flabbergasted voice—he realized who was calling. His panic turned into a whispered, sheepish confession: his wife would be back at any moment. It was Juliette's turn to be flabbergasted. The wife didn't like to travel, didn't mind him going by himself, and never asked questions. Juliette was fuming for having ignored her intuition. What were indeed the odds that such a charming man be still available at his age?

She ended the story by laughing off her deception. After all, she was "more perspicacious than someone working in the law enforcement field."

She also wondered why he and his wife stayed together until she thought of Mallick's wife. She likely suspected his double life, yet she always took him back.

Among her French travel companions on that trip, she befriended a couple from Paris.

I would meet them over dinner at her house after she was their guest in Paris. They enjoyed recounting their trip, including the episode of Juliette at risk of getting stranded outside Lima, at Jorge Chavez International Airport, or deported for using a false identity.

The confusion began when an airline ticket agent informed Juliette that she had already checked in. Time-consuming discussions led to a woman on the same flight and by the same name, except for her middle initial—a mistake that 'the woman by the same name' didn't bother correcting, not expecting a namesake on her flight. In this case, the odds of such a thing happening to Juliette were good; she was always a magnet for happenstances.

Sadly, Juliette's new friendship with the Parisian woman was illusory only.

When Juliette informed her of her illness, the woman promised to visit during her early chemotherapy treatments, but when the time came and Juliette was hospitalized, she wasn't interested in coming anymore. Instead, she complained about her non-refundable airline ticket from Paris to Geneva with EasyJet, a low-cost British carrier.

Juliette was bitterly hurt that the woman, a nurse, obviously didn't want to waste a long weekend on a doomed new friendship. Worse, she felt insulted not to be worth fifty euros anymore.

CHAPTER 34
A Long Conversation

BACK IN HER travel days, Juliette would have put a checkmark on her bucket list. We now put one on the list of her funeral arrangements. Strangely, it helps us end the day on a somewhat positive note—tomorrow is another day.

As her body begins its irreversible shutdown, death finds its insidious way into our conversations, coercing us to stay on the subject, as if reminding us that getting off would be the pretense that all is well. When we don't talk, I try to imagine what she thinks or feels. I only know what she shows or shares.

It's always on my mind that she asked me 'to accompany' her, yet I can't reconcile myself to what's best. If I am here when she dies, then her life will have ended. If she keeps on living after I've left, then she'll keep on suffering. As if reading my thoughts, she puts an end to my dilemma.

"Marie-Claude… I don't think I'll die… before you leave." She begins with my name, as we often do to deepen our closeness.

"I leave… in five days…" Guilt makes me hesitate. "I would like to be here when… uh—"

She interrupts: "I prefer that you came when you did… We still had a meaningful time."

I hear the past tense from the vantage point of her ending life.

"Let's face it… soon… I'll be half-conscious. I might not even know you'd still be here. I am so grateful that things are in place." I see the sadness in her eyes, then a faint glow of contentment.

I am grateful too, for Jim who insisted I didn't wait to be with her. I hold her hand, she immediately presses into mine as if I were a power outlet of a sort. I look into her brown eyes, losing myself in a gaze I never felt before. I scramble for something to say, anything to stop me from bursting into tears.

"I never thought of it before but… your eyes are like those of women from the Middle East… you know… that mysterious depth. Did you ever check your ancestry?" I am relieved to come up with a new thread in our conversation, unexpected for sure.

"Ah, my ancestors! I thought about that… I'm about to become one myself."

My spur-of-the-moment question and her equally unexpected answer make for a typical example of Juliette generating coincidence, so fitting that it ends my dazed state of mind. Do terminally ill patients often relate to their death as a passage into their ancestry? Juliette did.

"Are you still scared," I almost whisper, "as you were when we talked over the phone a couple of months ago?" Then I realize I am—almost naturally now—getting into *her conversation.*

She first responds with a sigh. "What I am the most afraid of… is to feel worse than I do now. I wish… I could fall asleep… and not wake up."

I now understand why it's often the wish of terminally ill people.

"I still wonder… how it will happen… you know?" She looks away, at the sky outside the window, anguish tormenting her face.

What do I say next?

"Perhaps you could think that uh… since we are born from this beautiful nature… when we leave this life, we are given back to this beautiful nature." The words come out of my mouth unforced, natural, mystifying.

"I never thought of it this way," she says.

I never thought of it like that before either and I am relieved that she doesn't challenge my reasoning.

Then I think of Sophie, who had—dare I say—decided to die. Yet that fatal moment of despair may never have happened had something or someone somehow interrupted that moment.

I forget what led Juliette to say one day that evidence showed that Sophie tried to free herself. As if the violent initial shock of hanging herself had jerked her out of that desperation. Hearing about it was so horrifying that I resisted the unbearable vision.

I often wondered whether Sophie's delayed, desperate survival instinct made it more intolerable for Juliette to think about her daughter's suicide. Or whether, in her mind, she could replace the word *suicide* with the word *accident*. I never summoned the courage to ask.

Sadly, imminent suicidal minds resist the thought that this very moment at the edge of the abyss shall pass. Still, it brings the question of whether that moment had passed before for Sophie, but not on that day. It may have, only too late. I come out of these disturbing thoughts as Juliette looks at me, again in a way that means, *keep talking!*

So, I do.

"There is a logic to remember. It even helped me before giving birth." I share how apprehensive I was until I thought, *yesterday it happened to some women, tomorrow it will happen to others, and today it's my turn*. Meanwhile, many women give birth every day in appalling conditions.

Feeling joined to all women by that collective and natural side of our destiny—giving life—helped me then. Today, I thought it would help me carry this conversation, but Juliette's raised eyebrows indicate that she doesn't see the analogy. I was giving birth. She is dying. And yet, the idea of our conjoined destiny as humans still holds. We come into this world, and we must eventually leave it, some of us sooner than others.

I try to think of other encouraging words, but what my heart feels, my mind doesn't know how to articulate. Then I think of my grandchildren who like to hear the same stories again, and again, each telling deepening their understanding. So, I repeat myself.

"Juliette… keep thinking about this… when we leave this life, we are given back to that beautiful nature. What comes with it cannot be ugly."

In retrospect, I wish I had elaborated on that beautiful nature with images of tropical fish, butterflies, and exotic birds, for example. The stunning harmony and precision of their colors and markings being nothing short of a miracle, scientifically based but still mind-blowing.

"You know… one can't deny the sacredness in the wonders of the natural world. For me, it's proof of a supreme power…

and whatever that power is, it escapes complete understanding. And yet, we are part of it." I had thought about this before, but voicing it suddenly resonates like a revelation.

"I hope I will think of this… and of you… when my time comes," I end this last thought with a sigh. Juliette seems to connect with what I said.

"Perhaps hell is our life on Earth… then death frees us… forever."

"I'll remember you said that."

"Whatever happens on the other side… I'll know it before you." She sounds the way little girls do when they try to outshine one another.

"Only you would think of it this way."

Acknowledging her humor was my way of saying *let's leave it at that for today*. I just expressed thoughts I have never voiced before, besides, what do I know about death? No one ever learned about it from someone who came back to describe how it was. Even if I had witnessed someone's last breath, I still wouldn't have experienced it. Death is a concept even for the dying.

"I must admit, it would help me to believe… in something." Hasn't she already said this? Never mind, she is unwilling to *leave it at that for today*. This puts me back in the moment, and of what came to my mind one night as I lay in bed unable to sleep.

"For me… what would help… is to know… that we'll be able to communicate… well… after—"

She interrupts: "We will… I promise… I will come back to haunt you!"

My gasped laugh relieves the oddness of our conversation, and her smile brings a much-needed lightheartedness. Smiling too, I get up to go to the bathroom and instinctively peek at the gap in the curtain drawn around the bed next to Juliette's. The woman is sleeping; she had cancer surgery two days ago, Juliette said. I wonder why patients next to Juliette never stay long, what was the type of *their* cancer, whether it was diagnosed very early, or too late for any treatment, and how their journey compares with Juliette's. This is still on my mind as I come out of the bathroom and find Juliette ready for me before I even sit down.

"You said you have… theories…"

I am still not used to her wanting to listen rather than talk. Plus, she now expects me to have something to say all the time. It's one thing to consider philosophical thoughts but quite another to share them with Juliette who hangs on my every word, giving to what I say the power to comfort or distress. And if I say nothing, Juliette may take my silence as a terrible acknowledgment of hopelessness.

And so, I tell her that what I read helped develop my theories, 'my unproven truth, my interpretable beliefs.'

Juliette doesn't make it easy for me to soothe her. She is an atheist—not believing that any god exists. At the same time, her questions suggest she is beginning to consider whether some God might exist after all—which would make her agnostic. Plus, I don't recall her mentioning the Golden Rule: "Do unto others as you would have them do unto you" (Matthew 7:12). Perhaps because that rule seems to have unfairly failed her. She had also brushed away the karma concept.

In brief, a person's action in this life determines their fate in 'another life.' However, karma has gone mainstream as our impatient society tends to attribute the punishing return of a bad action, or the reward of a good one, in the present time rather than in an uncertain reincarnated future.

I even considered whether Juliette rejected that notion, as a subliminal form of retaliation against Mallick. But he was an Indian Muslim—karma is a Buddhist and Hindu concept linked to reincarnation, and unthinkable in the Islam faith.

"This is the way I see it. Sometimes… not all the time. Remember… nobody knows for sure." I know that the convoluted subject I am about to try to explain is far from our habitual chatting, but my train of thought pushes me forward. "We know the body dies because it's tangible, but perhaps what's not tangible might not die. I know you don't want me to talk about the soul, so let's call it spiritual energy!"

"Huh?"

"That spiritual energy would continue to 'be' after death, but in another dimension."

She interrupts: "That's another thing I have trouble with. I mean… one thing turning into another!" She is challenging me more than I expected.

At that moment, a memory gives me another argument.

"Think about the water! Sometimes it's an ocean, sometimes a pond, or a river! Ah… but it can also be snow… or ice." I am getting her full attention. "What about a cloud or fog? It can even be invisible like the moisture in the air. It *is* one thing that can turn into another… and it still exists."

"How did you come up with… *this*?" I noticed the inflection.

"I heard something like it… somewhere."

I remember that such physical transformations helped me reconcile my intellect with my spirituality and only later would I remember where I had heard this.

It was in London, at the Speakers' Corner in Hyde Park, in the early nineties. A friend and I were walking by when, intrigued, we stopped to listen to the speaker of the moment.

He was claiming something like *God doesn't exist because it's invisible*. My friend then grabbed my arm, a stunned look on her face. Someone had just whispered in her ear, something about visible water turning into invisible moisture that is felt but not seen—alluding to God. She had turned in the direction of the voice so close to her ear, but no one was there. That person could have of course moved on quickly, but thunderstruck, my religious friend took it as divine intervention and I was left with a new perspective.

Our spiritual energy is a force that escapes understanding and that could perhaps leave us to join a universal 'presence' out *there*. It would be the *divine* that is felt even in the absence of faith in a doctrinarian God.

At the time, I hadn't watched the television show *Hollywood Medium with Tyler Henry*. His interpretations—of 'signs' from a departed—were both fascinating and troubling. Granted, it was a reality show with celebrities, with the associated bias. Yet Henry's revelations appeared to genuinely astound the participants. The messages received were of love or forgiveness, but also of suffering if a conflict wasn't resolved before that person died. Sometimes, they revealed secrets that led to closure for the participants. Sometimes, the departed was 'unwilling to establish contact.'

As I'd discover in the cover blurbs of books about mediums, clairvoyance is often disparaged as a scam, yet they give it traction in the context of psychic detectives—in law enforcement. Overall, there is evidence of a readership that is, if not deeply interested, at least troubled enough to want to know more about the subject.

As for *divine intervention*, the Internet is full of testimonials of such happy 'coincidences,' some troubling enough to challenge the intellect.

Tyler Henry's show would ease my concern about having shared my 'interpretable beliefs' with Juliette. Even outlandish thoughts are open to discussion when no proof to the contrary exists. A phenomenon can be undeniable yet scientifically unexplainable and is the reason for the *pseudoscience* label.

Drawn from the definition of pseudoscience in the Cambridge Dictionary, it relates to a system of thought, or a theory not developed in a fundamental scientific way. It doesn't mean there is no debate: Even the Stanford Encyclopedia of Philosophy admits that 'significant philosophical work must be done on the demarcation between science and pseudoscience.'

Years later, my 'interpretable beliefs' seemed less outlandish when I came across an article about Daniel Siegel—a professor of psychiatry at UCLA School of Medicine and the author of *Mind: A Journey to the Heart of Being Human*. In brief, Siegel and his multi-disciplinary scientist peers agree that our mind is not only the product of brain activity but exists beyond our physical self. The fact that electrocardiograms show emotions as brainwaves proves they exist in a physical sort of way. As I understand it, our spiritual energy would connect us beyond the earthly life of our brain.

Juliette is silent, expecting me to have more to say. It again crosses my mind that she may hope to pass while I am talking to her.

"People who say they died but came back to life also say

they felt peace, their mind becoming free as if nothing ever existed." The words *divine harmony* come to my mind, but I stop talking. I am entangled in concepts as unexpected, scattered thoughts keep coming. God or science? Philosophy might be open to interpretation, but religion demands unconditional belief in the Word of God.

Out the window, quietening white clouds float in the sky, and the thought of *divine harmony* reveals itself in a reconciliatory way, with the simple prayer for the soul: *Rest in peace*.

Juliette turns toward me, curling her body into the fetal position. She cups her cheek in the palm of one hand while the other one—hooked on to the IV—rests on her hip. She scrutinizes me as if assessing how much I believe in my *own* words. I know she might brush off my theories as tales.

"Are you sure that our spiritual energy… our soul… whatever… doesn't die with us?

Another question.

"I can't be sure since I can't prove it. But it often makes sense… at least to me. Besides, no one can be sure about such matters. That's why religion demands faith."

I don't share that much might change when the Big Bang Theory is elucidated, but I am likely conditioned by my dad's work environment, at the CERN.

I wish I had read, then, an article I'd come across later; it would have helped Juliette.

When the coral dies, it expels its colorful algal cells—the living energy that had thrived inside it. These algal cells then disintegrate in the water, and zillions of particles go on to exist somewhere else. The coral becomes a lifeless skeleton, like that of the human body. What if the mind was made of such cells, and going on to exist somewhere else when their keeper is gone?

Back to Juliette.

"Juliette… think of the body! We can see it and touch it… but not the mind, nor the spiritual energy. It's like ice versus moisture. The spirit isn't made of matter… it could go on to exist somewhere else. There is no proof either way."

Juliette then looks down, and she is so focused on my knees that I expect a comment about the color of my pants or their style. As the listener lying in bed, she looks as overwhelmed as me, the talker sitting at her bedside.

We both need silence but the occasional beeping from the patients' call buttons unsettles us.

Juliette turns on her back again and then closes her eyes, a faint smile on her lips, the kind that acknowledges something without great conviction.

I stay silent, relieved that she may fall asleep. I wait as still as a statue but have barely batted an eyelash when she looks at me.

"There are people I really don't want to see again."

It's the second time she is upset about this, and I am now upset too, for having said it. It didn't soothe her as I expected it would. I am neither a priest, nor a psychologist or a medium. I only have my heart and my consciousness to guide me—plus my 'interpretable beliefs.'

It's time to put an end to this conversation.

"You must be tired… no? We can talk more tomorrow. I'll stay here until you fall asleep."

"I am *not* tired… and I *don't* need to rest either… I'll have plenty of time for that where I'm going."

Bang! She is not leaving, not yet; every moment must count. I understand her implied request: *stay and keep talking!* And so, I go on, babbling until I get to a dead end.

"You know that mediums even work with forensic investigators… right? So—"

She interrupts: "Ugh… stop! You're giving me a headache." Now that she mentions it, I'm getting one too.

"It's getting late," I say after glancing at my watch. "I must go. I won't call you tonight, but I'll see you tomorrow… okay?"

"Don't be late! I may not be able to wait for you."

I see in her eyes that she enjoys having the last word, and I feel I am coming out of a long and grueling interrogation. I have nothing more to say, today.

CHAPTER 35
Dreaded News

EACH DAY BEGINS and then ends with uncertainty until I hear over our habitual morning phone call what I dreaded hearing all along.

"I'm getting transferred to the palliative care clinic," and after a split-second pause, she screams, "Tomorrow!"

Shocked and speechless that the postponement is over, I look out the window of my bedroom, at the mountain darkened by the somber green of the fir trees, at the chilled blue of the winter sky, at the scraggly, leafless trees of the neighborhood, and finally at the neighbors' bare garden below. Then I look back at the sky as if these visuals could help me process the news.

It has been a day-by-day delay that we hoped would last until the end, Juliette's end. Instead, Juliette is crushed and scared all over again. The news is an unrelenting reminder that she has no control over her life.

"Someone died… so… now it's my turn to go there and die too." Her voice is beyond spiteful.

My heart sinks from the weight of her bitterness and our combined sorrows. I understand her distress at yet another abandonment and her fear of yet another unknown. I hear myself say that she'll get even better attention *there*, where the staff will know how to guide her. I hope to give her something to think about until I am at her side. But I, too, am distraught by all that this transfer involves.

The nurses at the hospital were kind, supporting Juliette through the reality of her terminal illness. She endeared herself to them, earning their kindness and respect. Her departure to palliative care is hard for these nurses who were trained to promote health, prevent illness, restore health, and alleviate suffering. Compassion is all they can dispense now.

My aunt—the one who had the disastrous funeral—died in that hospital, and my cousins praised Head Nurse Nadège, who is also looking after Juliette. I haphazardly met her sister in her press and bookstore, in our village, after her conversation with a customer revealed who she was. From what I understood, Head Nurse Nadège's devotion to her patients affects her family life.

By the time I arrive at the hospital, Juliette is terrified. Her transfer will involve a forty-minute drive, by taxi-ambulance, and without the presence of a hospital staff member. In other words, it could be just her and a driver—someone she never met before.

She calms down when I tell her I'd never let her go alone. Then someone from the hospital administration comes to organize her discharge. Death row comes to my mind. The plan is for me to be at the hospital the next morning at 9:30. The rest of my visit goes by in a blur.

Before I leave, I lean over to kiss her forehead. She grabs my arm and looks into my eyes for something I can't or don't know how to give. It's hard to endure her stare and it crushes me to see her like this again. I manage a kind smile, but it's another wordless time.

It's not going to be all right; we both know it.

Then I remember Heidi's lesson. I must be in Juliette's *conversation*, even if it means a temporary lack of conversation. I must validate the way she feels. I must validate her fear. I must hold her desperate stare. I must accept all of it for what it is. It *is* the only way I can help.

"We knew it was coming... At least we won't be waiting for it to happen anymore... Everything is falling into place... Try not to fight it," I say as I cup her cheek.

She averts her eyes from my stare, her mouth crinkling into a wry smile as I get her unspoken comment: *You are not the one who will end up there*. I know I won't, but I feel it.

On my way out, I come upon Head Nurse Nadège in the hallway as if she was waiting for me. She asks how I am doing. She says Juliette cried a lot this morning when she told her about the transfer. I ask how much time she thinks Juliette has. I am sure she often answers that question.

"At least two weeks and at most four, but it could be sooner. The acid reflux is so strong she might even pass in her sleep. It could be suctioned, but Juliette refuses another paracentesis."

I don't remember how I got into my car until I arrive at the gate of the parking lot and can't go through. I can't because I don't have an exit ticket since I forgot to pay. I am angry, frustrated, and sad, and the only release is *Merde!* I am shocked; I normally curse in English, which sounds less reprimandable than in French. Today, I don't apologize for it.

Tomorrow will be a difficult day, and I am about to make it even more complicated.

I tell my parents I'll accompany Juliette to the palliative care clinic in the morning, and stupidly confirm I'll still join them, and my aunt and uncle, for the lunch we planned a week ago. Guilt is blinding me into expecting I can make the trip with Juliette and come back just in time for a family meal. I hope my parents offer to cancel. They don't, instead comparing the course of Juliette's illness to that of a friend who died from that cancer too.

Guilt is trapping me, and it's from my own doing.

CHAPTER 36

The Wait

I HAVEN'T SLEPT much, waking every hour or so to check my alarm clock. When I go downstairs, I don't want to talk and leave rapidly, telling my parents I'll see them for lunch.

At the hospital, a nurse assistant points to the visitors' lounge where I'll wait until Juliette is ready. Deep breaths help me stay calm until Head Nurse Nadège unexpectedly appears. Juliette wants to see me.

I notice uneasiness but we don't speak a word as I follow her. I know it's only the beginning of a dreadful day. She lets me in and opens the door to the en-suite bathroom. She then holds my interrogative stare—as if inviting me in.

And there is Juliette.

I freeze. I stop breathing. My throat tightens. My mind stalls. Juliette is standing by the washbasin, facing me. Unclothed for the most part.

Her emaciated body is of shocking color, not a jaundiced yellow as I understand it. It's darker, something like ocher, all over. Like that earthy shade in some of Van Gogh's paintings—after a chemical reaction dimmed the once glorious yellow pigment. That dimmed color of Van Gogh's sunflowers is now on my friend's skin—after chemotherapy, another type of chemical reaction, tarnished it too.

Long seconds go by as time stalls in silence. My open mouth feels dry. My eyes keep blinking as if it could help me think. No one moves until Juliette stretches her arms open. The way she did when she modeled new clothes.

"Meet the goddess of death!"

This is what *I* heard but is it what *she* said? She used the word *goddess*; of that I am certain. Did my mind put words to what I saw? Is there another goddess to allude to?

Her skin is the color of pancreatic cancer choking her bile ducks; it *is* the color of her approaching death. Her tight lips smile a defiant smirk. I get her silent cynicism—*can you believe this is me?*

She, Juliette, and her unbearable reality.

Her alien body is sickening to behold. It's skeletal like those of the women held in concentration camps, but her skin isn't grey. I can't wrap my mind around that odd ocher color, a brownish type of orange. It's the color of the tiles she had in mind and argued over in her mother's place in Provence.

I beseechingly glance at Nurse Nadège. Her worried eyes are locked on me, waiting. I take the appreciative stance that Juliette seems to expect. I barely know I am speaking, saying something like this: "*This is not who you are. This is just a box, and the woman I know isn't that box. The woman I know is beautiful, and a heck of a trouper.*"

"Yes, she is! I have rarely taken care of someone as strong as Juliette," Nurse Nadège says. "She is so realistic! And she has a good sense of humor too, and when it's least expected." She is relieved that I have overcome the shock and found the right things to say.

Juliette is looking at me. I read her face—sharing the sight of her body exorcised her *own* revulsion. She accepts her forthcoming death. Even the alienation from her *own self*.

Still dazed, I go back to the lounge, the vision of her jaundiced skin over her skeletal body stuck in my mind. I wonder whether it was iodine tincture, but it was all over her body. Like a bad application of tanning spray.

Will I ever forget this vision? My silent question hangs in my mind until the nurse assistant interrupts: "Juliette is ready."

Like an improbable team ready for action, Juliette and Nurse Nadège sit side by side on the edge of the bed. Juliette says nothing when I come in and stand in front of them, the three of us now waiting for the taxi-ambulance.

Juliette wears one of her winter jackets, now too large. She clutches her purse, her small duffel bag at her side. I hear them talk as if they were in another room. I dread what will happen next—accompanying Juliette to a place where she never wanted to go.

Juliette doesn't want the flowers that her visitors brought, but Nurse Nadège kindly insists, "They are part of your journey." Ten minutes go by, and we are still waiting.

Maybe there has been a mistake. Maybe she can stay. Meanwhile, Nurse Nadège stays with us as if nothing else matters. She knows Juliette needs her presence during this surreal wait. I do too. When Juliette thanks her for the kindness she bestowed on her, Nurse Nadège puts her arm around her shoulders and looks at me.

"Juliette had another big cry this morning. She also had a lot of questions, so we had a big chat." She implies that I should know this.

I then realize that Juliette never cried in front of me, not once, whereas I cried in front of her. I may not have been the recipient of her tears, but from that moment on, I stand as the guardian of her courage.

Juliette looks at Nurse Nadège timidly, like a little girl in need of her mother's encouragement. She asks whether she'll suffer as if she won't feel free to ask such questions *there*. It angers me that she can't stay *here*, going into an exile of a sort instead.

As I look at her, I see her not only physically but also mentally. I had learned to read her face and her mind. She won't have the strength to re-establish her identity as a terminal pancreatic cancer patient—with courage, humor, as well as vulnerability. She won't have time before her body further abandons her. She won't because this is 2014, and she isn't among the mere ten percent of cancer patients who survive five years.

Nurse Nadège rubs Juliette's back in small circles and replies that she still has a choice about the pain; it will depend on whether she eats or not. Food will keep her going but will exacerbate the pain too. Without food, her body will let go… Morphine will keep her comfortable…

This roadmap of her ending life is nearing the fundamental point of convergence. Her resolve will keep weakening until life surrenders.

It reminds me of what the dying mother of another friend said. From one moment to the next, she felt that as death approached, it stripped her of all that she had known and been, drawing her toward the nakedness in which she was born.

Forty nerve-racking minutes have passed when Juliette is

finally wheeled to the taxi-ambulance on the parking by the entrance. She hasn't been outside in months but doesn't take a deep breath of fresh air, doesn't look at the sky, or squint from the sun. Her impassive face looks straight ahead as if she were sleepwalking.

She wants to sit in the front of the car, a better place in her nauseated state. When she stands up from the wheelchair, it hits me that my friend has morphed into a caricature of herself. A frail old-looking woman in an oversized coat, her grizzled hair matted from not brushing it.

When we slowly exit the parking lot, I am still holding my breath. Even my thoughts are on hold. It's a sunny day, but I don't say that. It's the day we've been dreading for exactly one week. Rain or shine.

Juliette exchanges small talks with the driver, perhaps to blank out the unbearable first moments of her very last trip. I don't listen to their brief conversation, instead trying again to prepare for what happens next. And I don't know *what* that is.

Juliette was first hospitalized hoping surgery would be the solution to her bloated abdomen. But instead of returning home, she is going in the opposite direction. As if it's meant to further detach her from the life she knew. So she can face the elusive unknown ahead.

CHAPTER 37

A Convoluted Drive

THE DRIVER APOLOGIZES for his delay due to traffic jams in downtown Geneva. He informs us that he will bypass the main road to Pont du Mont-Blanc—the scenic bridge over the lake—and take the less-traveled neighborhood streets.

A few minutes into that drive, we are in Cointrin—the verdant suburb close to Geneva International Airport. Juliette says this is where they lived after moving from Paris to Geneva.

I knew about her young children's excitement when airplanes flew over before landing or after taking off. The airport wasn't busy then and its viewing deck was a local attraction. My dad sometimes took our family there as a Sunday afternoon outing and little did I know, then, that I'd become a regular air traveler.

I wonder how Juliette feels about this reminder of happier times when the driver's moaning interrupts my thoughts. The shortcut is not working. Roadwork has slowed the traffic into a bottleneck.

Another detour takes us through Grand-Saconnex, where people we know work for the European headquarters of the United Nations and its numerous agencies—Geneva counts more international organizations than any other city in the world. We are now one street over from where Juliette drove to work for more than twenty years, and where she met Mallick. She doesn't comment about what I see as another regrettable happenstance.

Unfortunately, this unwelcome 'sightseeing' of her life is not meant to be over. We drive by the International Center for Humanitarian Demining where Corinne is working at this very moment. Juliette doesn't look toward it nor speak. I sense that if she could, she would scream, the way she wanted after hearing she was terminally ill. Instead, her head deliberately veers to the opposite side, not even to me in the back seat, perhaps to avoid triggering nausea. I lay my hand on her shoulder. She knows I understand what's on her mind.

When we leave Avenue de France for yet another shortcut, she reaches for my hand, her fingers pressing into mine. She points to an adjacent street. "Mallick used to live on that street," she says in the narrative voice of an audio tour guide.

I don't know Mallick's address, but I am dumbfounded by yet another coincidence. Last October, Juliette said Mallick was the only man who made her feel cherished, despite his shortcomings. Unbeknownst to the driver, his unplanned itinerary turns into a sort of walk down memory lane, except that this is a drive, and it's real.

I sit on the edge of my seat, leaning forward to get closer and make her feel I am with her physically and emotionally. I am about to suggest this happenstance is a sign from Mallick, but she looks straight ahead, and when I press her shoulder again, I feel the stiffness.

I don't say anything; besides if I do this may be the moment she falls apart.

"Gridd-lo-oock," the driver moans again, apparently speaking to himself. "Haahr… can't go by Cornavin." He meant Gare de Cornavin, Geneva train station.

I can't snap out of *my* gridlock, the one that has overtaken my mind; can't even take a deep breath. I imagine the gripping tightness in Juliette's chest.

After forty minutes, we finally merge onto Quai du Mont-Blanc, but we are still on the lake's right bank. We drive by two of Geneva's historic hotels—Hôtel de la Paix and Hôtel Beau-Rivage—and several banks. Nonchalant visitors stand by the front windows of stores with the names of famous Swiss watchmakers: Rolex, Omega, Patek Philippe… On our left, the jetty of the Pâquis district ends with the lighthouse while the Alps hoist their snowy peaks in the distance. These familiar views suddenly feel alien, as if we no longer belong to the world out there. As if we are passing through to another time.

On this already convoluted drive, it's my turn to take a detour, unpredictable for sure. My gloomed mind brings up the tragic story of Empress Elisabeth of Austria and her life of suffering.

Sissi, as she was known, is remembered for her beauty, compassion, and life of hardships. In the late 1880s, she stayed incognito at Hôtel Beau-Rivage until she and her lady-in-waiting crossed the street—to board one of the boats that still cruise the lake—and an Italian anarchist stabbed her, enraged that the French royalty he planned to assassinate postponed his trip.

Sissi became famous for her tragic death after having lost a young daughter, and then her adult son the crown prince, while more tragedies plagued the rest of her family. She also spent hours grooming her opulent knee-length hair. A story that Juliette likely knew of, and an obsession she would have understood.

At last, we access Pont du Mont-Blanc where multicolored flags indicate that some international organization is in session. On the right is Île Rousseau—the islet named after the philosopher Jean-Jacques Rousseau who was born in Geneva. His statue stands on a tall pedestal, but the café in the domed pavilion where Juliette and I often spent our lunch break has shut.

At the left end of the bridge, I glance at the National Monument that commemorates the reunification of Geneva with Switzerland. Two women named *Republic of Geneva* and *Helvetia* hold one a sword and the other a shield, turning forever their backs to France—to which they had belonged—looking instead to the north, toward Switzerland—their new future.

Juliette and I are going in the same direction, but the association ends here.

Immediately after, we come upon L'Horloge Fleurie—the clock flower bed is the symbol of the illustrious Swiss horology industry; it always shows the precise time, but we drive by too fast for me to notice it.

Our silent drive-by continues with Le Jardin Anglais—the English garden. In the mid-1800s, flowing, romantic English gardens were preferred to the formal, structured *jardins à la française*.

When the driver then merges onto Quai Gustave-Ador, Juliette turns her head to look at Geneva's iconic landmark, Le Jet d'Eau—Europe's highest fountain, and a fluke. The first one was built to regulate the water pressure of the nearby hydraulic plant, but after it became a public attraction, it was rebuilt here. Juliette likely remembers bringing her young children here. We all did. And perhaps she strolled incognito along the quay on a romantic summer evening with Mallick.

The Jura Mountains are now on our left. In their foothills, a string of villages populates the Pays de Gex, where Juliette lived and where I was born.

We are only halfway to our destination.

Juliette sits motionless as if she were under hypnosis for this anguishing transition. And I am still overcome by incredulity that this trip is really happening. My breath is short, and I bite the side of my lips. I wish someone else was with us, someone who could fill the oppressive silence.

Juliette will never again see the scenery that unfolds beyond the car window, and I can't imagine she is not thinking about it too. My hand holds hers from the back seat, and both are cold. I don't have to press into hers; she is gripping mine. We are going through this ordeal together. No one should ever have to go through it alone.

Geneva is 'our' city—despite it not being in France—and Switzerland's second largest, after Zürich. Despite improvements, traffic must funnel its way onto Pont du Mont-Blanc, which is the main access across the croissant-shaped lake, fed by the Rhône River—from Montreux on the northeast to Geneva on the southwest. The Rhône begins as an alpine glacier and ends in Camargue, near Arles, a one-hour drive from Marseille.

I am attached to Geneva's familiar landmarks, perhaps the reason I feel drawn to turn back and look at the elevated Old Town—towered over by Cathédrale St. Pierre. In earlier years, Juliette and I often had lunch there, then browsed the quaint shops alongside the cobblestone streets to the fortifications.

There, the Monument de la Réformation stands as the memorial to early Protestant leaders such as John Calvin, his strict leadership having imprinted an everlasting sense of discipline and conservatism upon Geneva. In fact, after living here for several years, my British-Canadian husband still says, "In Switzerland, things are either compulsory or forbidden." But for this reason, the citizens know what to do, how to do it, and when.

We drive by the exit for La Gradelle, in Chêne-Bougeries, the Geneva suburb where Jim and I were married and where our family once lived. Then we come upon Cologny, an enclave with luxurious properties anchored on a hill overlooking the lake.

In the coastal town of Vésenaz, the driver leaves Route de Thonon for Route d'Hermance, toward our destination. That our next turn will be our last squeezes my stomach into a growl that reminds me that I was too tense to eat breakfast.

None of us spoke a word since we left Geneva.

Moments later, the road sign for Collonge-Bellerive appears more like a threat than a geographic destination. We arrive in the Swiss town where the University Hospital houses the palliative care clinic. Even a seemingly endless trip comes to an end.

Juliette reaches again for my hand. She still doesn't speak. I again press hers and barely hear myself comment on the quiet surroundings. She likely didn't expect to hear much else from me.

Centuries-old houses with traditional and sturdy architecture line the main street. Some have transitioned into apartments and restaurants; others are still farmers' homes. In the summertime, red and white geraniums—the national colors—brighten the traditional wooden shutters and planters on the windowsills. But on this wintry day in February, the neutral colors of the dormant farmland and gardens blend into a monochromatic, spiritless scenery.

A white road sign with a blue capital H for *Hospital* indicates our exit. Chemin de la Savonnière, number 11. I look out the car window and up to the cerulean sky where crows zigzag in a black pattern. Like vultures over roadkill. Gloom is overtaking me.

Marianne! The sight of the parking lot suddenly brings me back to reality. Juliette is unaware that Marianne is waiting for me in this parking lot while I help her settle in. My two friends haven't seen each other in decades, and Marianne has avoided hospitals since Jean-Paul died in one. Marianne is here to drive me back to Geneva, from where I'll take a bus to the hospital where my car is parked.

All of this so I could be on time for my family lunch.

Lunch! The word strikes my mind like lightning in the sky. How am going to make it on time after our delay? I already know that it's impossible. I tried to call Marianne when we were first delayed, but my flip phone got no signal. I now have no idea where Marianne parked her car, and she must wonder why we didn't arrive almost two hours ago. She may not even be here anymore.

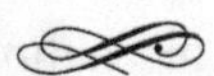

MARIANNE LIVES IN France, a ten-minute drive from the Swiss

palliative care clinic. My best friends, however, never cared much for each other.

Marianne was the more reluctant one, perhaps because of Jean-Paul's reservations about Juliette. I never understood the reason for a reticence that was not reciprocal. Juliette appreciated his intellect and good company.

After the publication of *The ABCs of Jazz*, Jean-Paul embarked on a career at a Swiss but French-speaking radio station, where he celebrated his five-hundredth show a few months before he died.

Over his thirty-year career, he provided television commentary for the Montreux Jazz Festival. He interviewed legendary French singers, musicians, and actors, commemorating their lives, and recording their memories and words of wisdom. And most impressive, some would say perplexing, he was the only radio host known to use *l'imparfait du subjunctive*—the imperfect of the subjunctive; this extinct English subjunctive mood used in romance language literature, and at the *Académie Française*—the bastion of the French tongue.

Jean-Paul spoke the traditional language of journalism with ease, but not in a casual conversation with Juliette. The combination of her guardedness and insistent demeanor might have intimidated him unless it irritated him.

Jean-Paul was a good friend whose judgment I trusted. We'd listen to music in the basement: he, puffing on his pipe; me drawing in the minty taste of thin Davidoff cigars; Marianne tapping to the beat and silently resenting the smoke. Jean-Paul prepared the audio part of his radio shows in this audio room almost entirely lined with some 20,000 vintage records and CDs.

How strange that Juliette and Marianne are my two best

friends, each living on opposite sides of Lac Léman, at the foot of mountains facing each other. And yet they were both born in Paris.

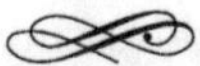

THIS *IS* IT—THE end of my friend's last trip.

I open the door of the taxi-ambulance to the disquieting cawing of crows. A *murder of crows*, they are called. The old myth of their symbol of the afterlife is hard to miss; never mind that they are now deemed the carriers of enlightening messages. Today, I know what they mean to us.

Juliette has already opened the door of the car when I get to it, and she refuses my help. She looks robotic, resigned… wretched. She reluctantly sits in the required wheelchair, and I wheel her toward the lobby where the automatic doors open like threatening jaws. This is no *Jonah and the Whale* story, though. Juliette won't be saved, swallowed instead by a wicked illness that knows no redemption. My mind stalls as we cross the threshold of two worlds: life on one side and death on the other.

Marianne! She is standing at the back of the lobby, flowers in hand. Her unexpected presence immediately relieves the tension that clung to me since we left the hospital. Unsure of what to do, she waits until I walk over after leaving Juliette at the registration desk. She hasn't seen Marianne yet and may not have recognized her immediately. When I reintroduce them, Juliette looks pleased by her presence.

In the back of my mind, I hear Marianne's words after Jean-Paul died: *Death is monstrous. It takes someone you love and never gives them back.*

A female attendant greets us. I am taken aback that a terminally ill patient in a visibly strained state should go through a lengthy registration process. I quickly change my mind; Juliette isn't whisked in as if she didn't have a say in this.

The attendant smiles, addressing us as *mother and daughter*. Juliette takes it almost well. "I am not her mother, we are friends… but I am thirteen years older. I know… I don't look my best today." I hear the dash of annoyance in her attempted humor.

The attendant quickly makes amends. "A daughter usually accompanies her mother—you must be very close friends." This is not the best of all possible starts. Somewhat embarrassed, Marianne points to the sitting area where she'll wait.

"What is the name of your husband?" the attendant asks Juliette.

"I am divorced."

"I still need his name."

"Dimitri Volvinsky."

"What is his address?"

"He is deceased."

"How many children do you have?"

She hesitates. "Three."

"What are their names and addresses?"

Juliette has responded matter-of-factly to the attendant's string of direct questions, but she hesitates again. She gives her oldest daughter's and son's full name and address, then waits. The attendant looks up, expecting her answer.

"My youngest daughter… is deceased."

"What was her name?"

"Sophie Volvinsky."

"What are the names of your mother and father?"

These unflinching, necessary, yet polite questions prod at Juliette's past in a purgatorial way. As if her life must be stated in black on white, one last time. As if her answers are recorded for an evaluation of how she lived her life unless it's to remind her of what she lived through. Her approaching death is enabling unwelcome questions that she must face one more time. It's no longer a confession; it's not quite atonement since she was also a victim, but she must still lay her cards on the table, faces up. This last question likely reignites her resentment of her father while she receives it as the last scornful 'sign' from her mother.

I stroke Juliette's shoulder, slowly but firmly. This expiating process blanked her face, but I can still read it: *capitulation*.

Then, she is curious about her new surroundings as soon as we turn away from the registration desk.

She leans forward as I push the wheelchair to follow the assistant to the elevator, down to the palliative care ward, and then along a hallway. We have entered a vacuum. I barely breathe. There is no hospital smell. The ceiling light has a ghostly white glow. The only sounds are my muffled steps and the faint wheeling of the chair. Everything is eerily neutral. Silent.

When the door opens, I expect a confined hospital room; instead, a glass wall rises from the natural surroundings. A heavy curtain separates the spacious room into two sections and faint voices indicate that the patient has a visitor. I feel a complicated interconnectedness, between the natural and the supernatural, the living and the dying.

The assistant helps Juliette lie in bed, then I place her personal effects in her closet and on the table in front of the glass wall. I ask for vases. The flowers that Nurse Nadège convinced her to take along now blend with the lawn where tiny white daisies announce the coming of spring.

When we are alone, and in her still matter-of-fact way, Juliette wants me to 'sort out' what I put in the closet. A book that was a gift must go with things that she 'doesn't need nor want.'

"*Voilà*!" she says, opening her arms to acknowledge her new space.

I know. This is *it*.

I bring a chair close to her bed. I must re-establish our connection. Make her feel safe. I hold her hand, hoping she feels the love. Sadness washes over me. Uncontrollable tears spill over and run down my cheeks. It's too late to hide them. I know I feel what I feel. It would be odd if I didn't. But I am supposed to be the strong one here. Juliette looks at me intently, as she has done so many times since her diagnosis.

"Remember… I have no choice." Her gentle yet assertive tone makes me regret my weakness even more. I admire her strength. Then, I wonder whether she is still afraid of death.

"I'm not afraid of dying anymore," she says as if it was her turn to read my mind. There is no anxiety in her voice. The fear of ending up in this palliative care clinic was more terrifying than being here physically. "But I'm still afraid of dying in pain." Pain has been another fear.

I remind her of Head Nurse Nadège's words: "Painkillers will keep you comfortable." I can't say the word *morphine* yet; in her case, it will be the last treatment. Then two doctors, a nurse, and an assistant come into the room and ask for privacy. I can't leave just yet.

"I am going to join Marianne and will come back later."

"Tell her she can come too!"

Marianne barely holds it together when she sees I've cried.

She is shocked by what cancer did to Juliette's appearance. This no longer shocks me, but what suddenly does is remembering that I still haven't let my parents know that I won't join them for lunch. I dread calling, anticipating my mother's disappointment or disapproval. When I do, she "understands;' my dear aunt likely had something to do with it.

"Juliette seemed pleased to see me," Marianne says. "It made me forget my fear of hospitals.

Fifteen minutes later, Juliette welcomes us back with a smile. She comments on her new surroundings and looks appeased. She tells Marianne she often thought of her after Jean-Paul died.

"I called you sometime later, but I felt I was disturbing you."

I remember Juliette telling me this. I now wonder how Marianne will react to Juliette's typical candor.

"I wasn't quite myself for a long time. I'm sorry, I don't remember, but it was nice of you to think of me."

A nurse comes in. It's time for us to leave. Marianne offers to come back since she lives close by, and I remind Juliette that tonight is the beginning of the weekend.

"Remember… I'm not coming tomorrow or Sunday—your family is. I'll see you on Monday. It has been an exhausting day… You did well. I'm proud of you." She smiles one of her tired smiles. I lean in to kiss her forehead. There is no I.V. in the way.

There is no more treatment.

I walk out of the hospital as if I am fleeing. My lungs once more fill with fresh air then exhale the trembling sensation inside me. A friend is waiting to take me home to the rest of my life after I took another to the end of hers. It's impossible not to think it.

CHAPTER 38

One Day at a Time

I AM SPENDING the weekend with my parents, chatting, relaxing in my bedroom during their afternoon nap, and collecting my thoughts. Relatives and friends drop by and catch up on news over coffee in the morning, tea in the afternoon, and perhaps an aperitif later in the day. That's why our family home's nickname is *Café de la Gare*—from the long-gone café on that street to the former train station. I often miss this way of life that also keeps my parents engaged in their old age.

During the nice season, they all sit in the veranda, but on wintry mornings, my dad prefers the kitchen to the living room, which frustrates my mom who is cooking.

When I help her prepare lunch—still the main meal in France—I hear a dash of irritation as she asks about Juliette. Then at the end of the day, my dad beats about the bush before asking whether I'll watch *C Dans l'Air* (*It's in the Air*), a television talk show about national and international headlines. We usually watch it before dinner, but it hasn't happened often during this visit. I am drained and need a bit of a quiet transition when I get back from visiting Juliette.

I understand that my time with Juliette is affecting our time together. When I address the tension, my mom goes on the defensive and my dad escapes to the living room. I get that unpleasant but familiar feeling of being pulled in opposite directions. Pleasing everyone is impossible—*this* I know—but whatever I do never feels as if it's enough. It's *my* perception of the situation, but it's real to me. As a result, that perception often leads to what I think are other people's expectations of me.

The fact that I live far away makes our time together precious, but this is one case when my perception is not distorted. My friend needs me more than my parents do right now. I see a similarity with the jealousy of Juliette's mother, that of our natural possessiveness when someone else takes precedence over what we consider our own.

I also find myself paying more attention to my parents' home, dreading the time when this will come to an end too. Juliette never mentioned hers again after we brought a selection of her clothes. She completely estranged herself from what used to wholly ground her. Perhaps her mind has organically let go of what isn't serving her anymore, clearing the way for the 'tunnel of light' that Corinne wrote about.

I also think of her desolate appearance, of how she gently pats her hair now completely matted into the appearance of a felt headdress, then arranges it on each side of her face, likely for the familiar sensation it provides. She still hasn't let anyone comb it. She hangs on to it, perhaps less as a little victory and more as a substitute for a soothing baby blanket.

She avoids mirroring surfaces because of the frightening 'alien' who always stares back at her. My beautiful friend has morphed into the appearance of a mummy. Weight loss froze her face as if her womanhood left with the vanished flesh. When I rub moisturizer on her arms, her skin seems to want to slide off her bones. Her lifeless hair, her shadowy face, and her skeletal body are all but vile messengers. Even her hands have lost their character.

Juliette is like the blueprint on an architect's table—lines that define a shape. And I come to a sarcastic conclusion: it's best to die in good health, although after a long and well-lived life.

CHAPTER 39

Serendipity, Destiny, Fate, Happenstance

JULIETTE IS SURRENDERING her body to cancer and stories to me. As if she must share more than the stories that defined her until now. As if I must know more, but I am not sure why. I think of this when I retreat to my bedroom in the evening.

I look for something to read in the basket at my bedside. I find airline inflight publications—for travel articles; French magazines that my mother saved for me, to reconnect with French pop culture; and inspirational books, to relax my mind into a good sleep. I find a book I read a long time ago and planned to get reacquainted with: *La Force de l'Âge* (*The Prime of Life*) by Simone de Beauvoir.

I retrieved it on a previous trip, from the small former kitchen on my bedroom floor, which I'd turned into a study—with a sink—and the cupboards into a secret library—with an eclectic collection of books, in French.

As I skim and peruse the pages, one of de Beauvoir's statements retains my attention, and I ponder whether it would be true that we cannot know our story, we can only tell it.

I take this well-timed encounter as the gift of serendipity, meant to help me understand Juliette through her stories.

Aside from pioneering feminism, the self-absorbed existentialist author hadn't inspired me much in this memoir. She could tell her story since she wrote the book, but she shows no awareness of her annoying sense of entitlement. In that sense, she didn't know herself.

During World War II, she often counted on the generosity of friends, and their friends, and acquaintances as well to get her through her difficulties, yet she had options, had she been willing to rely more on herself.

Other than for Jean-Paul Sartre—her journalist/political activist/lover—captured by the Germans, her only concern was herself. In that sense, she abided by his train of thought as the leader of the French existentialist philosophy: "[S]he gave meaning to h[er] own life by seeking to please [her]self, first."

In any case, de Beauvoir raised in my mind the question: *how do our stories relate to who we are?* Evidently, our stories seem to give that perspective to our readers or listeners only.

I would find such an example in the nail-biting novel *The Nightingale*. Inspired by a true story, Kristin Hannah depicts the lives of two French sisters during World War II. Both risk their lives every day: the oldest in her village, the youngest as a member of *La Résistance* against Nazi Germany.

Their selfless actions trample upon danger with courage and shrewdness, which they didn't know they possessed. Love keeps them going: one for her family and friends, the other for the fleeting but unforgettable romance that sustains her patriotic fight beyond the tolerable.

Their stories reveal who they are—yet again not to them. In that sense, wartime was their fate, and bravery in their destiny. It is so for heroes; they know the story of their 'heroic' acts, but they don't relate to their heroism, downplaying it as something they had to do instinctively. In that sense, Hannah's book illustrates de Beauvoir's statement.

In turn, each of Juliette's stories leads me to discover more of who she is.

But what she keeps calling *my destiny* I call *her fate*. I associate *fate* with negativity and darkness. After all, the opening sentence: *On that fateful day*… isn't the introduction to a happy outcome.

The guilt from her daughter's suicide was Juliette's fate, as was questioning whether leaving her husband sooner or staying married longer could have prevented her death, or her son developing a mental disorder. The lack of a bond with her mother was also her fate and so perhaps the shared hostility with her oldest daughter. As for her unsecured relationship with Mallick, I am not sure whether it was fate or destiny.

The image of a puzzle again comes to my mind. By revisiting with me the significant events of her life, Juliette is giving me more of its components. It's now up to me to figure out how they fit together to get the whole picture.

It might be the reason, out of the blue one day, that Juliette talks about her mother again. I thought I already knew why they were so conflicted—her mother ignoring the scene of Juliette accusing the salesman of abuse was reason enough. I hear that Juliette's mother was seven years old when she lost her own mother and was thereafter rejected by a stepmother. I also hear it as if it should reveal the clue to a riddle.

Women deprived of love in childhood can of course become affectionate mothers, but Juliette's mother was evidently not one of them. Sadly, her *own* inner conflicts would likely explain her cantankerous character, and her inability to connect with her daughter.

Why had Juliette never told me of her mother's childhood? I imagine it was too painful to accept that she was repeating the cycle. I would be reminded of this by an article in a French magazine—*Inexploré, 2019*—in which Anne Ancelin Schützenberger, the founder of psychogenealogy, explains that *when we don't understand how our history fits in our life, we are not free to make choices.*

As for Corinne, I am not sure whether she knows of her grandmother's hardships, or her family's intergenerational traumas.

When I ponder Juliette's life, I still worry about not seeing the whole picture and forgetting to say something that could soothe her last days—that I would understand it too late.

Another book would bring another instance of serendipity and later reconcile me with that worry.

In *Truth and Beauty*, Ann Patchett shares her friendship with Lucy Grealy, who lives her entire life disfigured by cancer, challenged by surgeries, and defiant of her destiny. Patchett did much more for Lucy than I ever did for Juliette, yet she still has one regret when her friend 'unexpectedly' dies. Patchett laments her friend's belief that the 'most basic rules of life' didn't apply to her. She felt it was her mistake to believe it too.

From Patchett's words, it dawned on me that in true friendship as in true love, and because nothing ever seems to be enough, there should be no such question as *what more could I have done?*

Then happenstance keeps happening. This time, it's with an article in *Science et Avenir—Science and Future*. After forty years, my dad's subscription yielded some 'worth keeping' magazines in unusual places—the attic, the cellar.

The article is about CERN—the European Center for Nuclear Research, previously mentioned—and the long-awaited experiment of smashing particles in the Large Hadron Collider to identify the Higgs boson: the last particle needed to complete the Big Bang theory of the origin of the universe. CERN confirmed the existence of the Higgs boson—on March 14, 2013.

What does this have to do with Juliette? you may ask.

First, it happened on Juliette's birthday, exactly one year before her death. *Second* is rather bewildering.

This collider—an underground ring with a circumference of 26.7 kilometers (16.6 miles) and at a depth ranging from 50 to 175 meters (164 to 574 feet)—encompasses a territory not only agricultural but also commercial and residential, and among which is Juliette's home, and what's more, the cemetery where she'll be laid to 'rest in peace.'

Never mind that this collider is deemed 'the Jurassic Park for particle physicists, and 'the first big step to unraveling the creation of the world—as per the article *The Beginning* in Bloomberg Business Week, March 30, 2012. To the very end, Juliette never failed to be part of yet another almost unbelievable but true story.

CHAPTER 40

Family and Friends

THIS JOURNEY WITH Juliette gives me a deeper appreciation for my life, for the odds that I could be the one dying. I share my thoughts with Jim on the telephone every night to unload my heavy heart. I also email my children in Canada and the United States, who have met Juliette.

> *For Juliette, things are following their unavoidable course. [...] I have experienced moments of emotional challenge. [...] All I can say is that it has been sad and yet helpful in some unexpected ways. Juliette wants to discuss everything in very realistic and truthful ways. It has been a life lesson.*
>
> *It's particularly tough for Corinne, who has a difficult relationship with her mother. She is so exhausted after six months of this. [...] I had a very good connection with her from the start, which helped a lot. She was still very angry with her mother but trusted my understanding of their relationship.*
>
> *Of course, nobody is perfect, not even, perhaps especially not a mother. [...] There are reasons that explain how we have become who we are. They needed to make peace so neither had regrets from things left unsaid and unforgiven.*

I have paced myself the whole time, although I am with her almost every day. I stay away on weekends, so I don't infringe on family time, and we talk on the phone mornings and evenings.

I am ready to return home on Wednesday because no one knows how long she will live, although I can't imagine her surviving much longer. I wish I could be here, but I have done what she asked, and her last days should be with her family. She is very grateful that I could come now rather than later.

I am sad, but also happy to be able to go back to my life (…) It's a blessing that losing my friend is balanced by the birth of a healthy baby in our family.

Congratulations to the new great-aunts and uncles!

Lots of love to each of you.

Mom, Butch, Nana

Butch is the nickname that stuck with my then two-year-old step-granddaughter—and now my step-great-grandson's mother—after she heard my husband's imaginative term of endearment one day.

I needed to share my sadness with my family and read their words of support the next morning. The situation helped them put their daily annoyances in perspective, they said. They reminded me that all I could do was to be with my friend. I now realize that my emotions took over and that nothing mattered but what I was experiencing. From that, I remind myself that a patient ear is the best encouragement to anyone. As I connect my words to those of my family, I know I am experiencing more than the end of my friend's life.

I am on a journey of self-discovery.

Sadly, shortly after Juliette would die, my daughter-in-law lost her own friend from an aggressive type of ovarian cancer. What she shared gave me another perspective, that of my experience being more about sadness whereas hers was also about revolt. And yet, I, too, revolted against her friend's fate that didn't grant her the legitimate right to raise her children. I would argue that both our friends feared death, only in different ways. Juliette's fear was somewhat natural at her advanced age. She could talk about it. *We* could talk about it. It wasn't so for that young mother who refused to talk about it, even with her husband.

One can only imagine that the excruciating sorrow of leaving their two little girls took over her fear of dying. She refused to let her illness hijack the time she still had with her family, perhaps to protect them from that fear, and protect herself, too. As the mother of young children, my daughter-in-law could relate to her friend's tormenting yet repressed pain, a pain more visceral than mine ever was about Juliette. The insight, here, is that one must indeed measure one's challenges against those that take precedence; sometimes it's just the natural order of things.

This made me think of parents who lost a child, of young couples in which a spouse died, or anyone who lost a young family member. I lost my friend but came to a reckoning: although Juliette could have lived another twenty years, at least she lived most of one's life expectancy.

Friends suggest I watch films with Juliette, listen to music, read to her, look at photographs, and "share laughter and tears." One friend hopes that "Juliette is of the mind that this life isn't the end." Another writes, "We will all follow."

I welcome my friends' support yet most advice on providing companionship to a dying person is unrealistic. Such soothing pastimes may be possible in the early stages of an illness, but Juliette's discomfort and painkillers aren't conducive to enjoyment. The last and only time I saw Juliette enjoy herself, and momentarily forget her illness, was on one of my early visits in the hospital.

I had come with my mother, who Juliette was expecting that day. Her son was there too. I hadn't seen him since I bought the merry-go-round painting, perhaps ten years prior.

Our arrival was met by Juliette's state of excitement, and it wasn't toward us since she barely greeted us, somewhat embarrassing her son. She was watching on television the women's ice hockey final of the 2014 Winter Olympics Games in Sochi, Russia.

Her eyes riveted on the screen, she demanded that we 'hold still and watch' the last three minutes of the Canadian women in overtime play for the gold medal. She then cheered Canada's 3–2 victory over the United States, and with great exuberance imagined Jim—my Canadian hockey-fanatic husband—cheering too. She had watched the game from the beginning and even knew that this Canadian women's victory matched the record for Olympic gold medals held by Russian men. She even remembered watching the previous Winter Olympic Games, in 2010 in Vancouver, aware that most of our family was together for this exciting event in our city.

I never saw Juliette watch television after that day.

Would she have called it *destiny* or *fate*, had she known she would be in this hospital four years later? Fortunately, she enjoys listening even if she is no longer the prolific storyteller.

CHAPTER 41
The Lawn Daisies

ON THIS EARLY Monday afternoon, the traffic is unusually slow in Geneva. It gives me too much time to think that I'll leave in three days. I haven't seen Juliette over the weekend and wonder how she feels as she copes with her move to the clinic. What else will we talk about? I have nothing more to say and yet keep worrying about what might be left unsaid.

The queues at the red streetlights also give me time to look at the people and storefront windows along the way. Over the years, the stores mirrored the increase in Geneva's population diversity. Some have been here for decades—Swiss people like traditions. Most have been converted into shops for ethnic food, the latest electronic gadgets, vaping devices, tattoo parlors, and other specialties that didn't exist when I lived here; restaurants followed suit, too.

As I finally merge onto the lake's left bank, I get an expanded view of the Jura. Its geological singularity, straight up above the village, is akin to a familiar feature on a face. It's 'my mountain,' never mind that it stretches into an arc of over 225 miles (360 kilometers) from the Rhine to the Rhône rivers. It's always beautiful with its green forested flank—Jura comes from the Celtic word *forest*—and today, it's magnificent with the white layer of fresh snow against the crisp blue sky. Compared to the precipitous summits of the Alps across the valley, the roundness of the Jura seems to invite hikers on her lap, never mind its steep incline.

I drive through the Swiss town of Collonge-Bellerive, noticing people who walk out of a *boulangerie-pâtisserie*—a bread and pastry shop—some holding a box, some a loaf of bread, or both. For a split second, the thought of getting croissants crosses my mind, but I am not visiting Marianne in her home. I am visiting Juliette at the clinic and food is no longer part of her life. Guilt chases the whiffs of freshly baked goods in my mind.

When I get out of the car, the fresh air recharges my emotional battery. I am calm as I walk into the lobby, yet it dawns on me that even in Switzerland anyone may enter a hospital freely, perhaps even more so than in some other public places. I take the elevator and head to Juliette's room without anyone asking me where I am going or what I am doing, here.

In Juliette's bedroom, I immediately notice that all the flowers are gone, even Marianne's. Were they too painful a reminder of her garden? Of funerals? Perhaps it was her reason for wanting to leave them behind. Perhaps they simply died.

I also notice lawn daisies in a glass on her nightstand, the same that polka-dot the grass outside her window; I wonder how *these* ended up here. I can no longer guess from Juliette's face what's on her mind, but when I mention the *pâquerettes*, she has a story to tell.

Yesterday, Juliette's son visited with his girlfriend, and Corinne with her family, and it happened to be Grandmother's Day, a French 'tradition' that began in the late 1980s.

"Can you believe it? No flowers... and no mention of it."

"Hum... I'm not familiar with this celebration. We don't have it in America, and it didn't exist when we lived here."

"I was *so-oo* disappointed." I hear anger more than disappointment.

As I would later hear from Corinne, on the way to the clinic, no florist or grocery store was open—on Sundays, in Switzerland. Uncertain of whether Juliette knew what day it was, no one mentioned it. But Juliette knew. She didn't need special flowers, pointing to the *pâquerettes* on the lawn instead, and asking her grandchildren to pick some for her.

A nurse assistant interrupts her recounting and comments on the "pretty flowers" in the glass. I am as surprised by the kind comment as I am by Juliette's answer.

"They are from my grandchildren, for Grandmother's Day."

Juliette's reaction is not so much about that special day as it is about showing that her family cares. Perhaps it's the implicit need to assess her identity in this community new to her, as she did when she told the hospital nursing staff that I came from North America to be with her. It set her apart from the other patients.

What surprises me, though, is a staff member engaging in a personal comment. Unlike at the hospital, the clinic staff only presented a routine devoid of compassion on the day we arrived. Something Corinne would eventually comment on before I did.

...Back to the failed Grandmother's Day celebration.

I wonder what to say since Juliette is now always eager to hear me speak. But she has much on her mind today.

She talked to her family as if she was making an announcement. She wanted them to understand the gravity of the moment, that it could be the last time she talked to all of them at once.

To set herself up before sharing that announcement, she asks me to prop up the pillows that never seem to support her comfortably. Then, as the protagonist of her story, an actor or orator, she raises her chin with conceit and begins to speak to me like to an imaginary audience.

I am stunned by her sudden assertive vitality and wonder whether it's a side effect of the painkillers. Still distracted by her behavior, I only hear the main points.

She told her son she was giving him her car, and her daughter her diamond ring. Her son asked permission to sell the car—unable to afford the insurance. Corinne didn't tell her mother what she would tell me later.

She was upset to be 'stuck' with an eye-catching ring that she wasn't allowed to sell and would never wear. She also referred to her mother's 'performance' as the 'delusional way' in which she addressed them, wondering about a side effect of the medication, too.

Nothing was ever simple in Juliette's family circle.

Juliette didn't want Corinne to sell the diamond ring because it symbolizes Mallick's love. She wants it to become a family heirloom, something to remember her by.

"Mallick was the only man who made me feel cherished." She's said this before, but her tone of voice solemnizes her statement. I nod, solemnly too.

Juliette is thirsty and asks for Coca-Cola, and there is none. Sips of it are all that her body tolerates, plus crushed ice cubes of pineapple juice. The nurse assistant has no explanation for the lack of Coca-Cola but informs me that it's available at the cafeteria. Shocked by her attitude, I say I evidently must get it myself.

On my way to the cafeteria, I walk by the nurses' lounge and since the door is open, I inquire about the Coca-Cola shortage. One nurse then gets up, asks me to wait, walks to a room across the hall, returns shortly thereafter, and hands me a can. Perplexed, I thank her without further comment.

Another incomprehensible attitude has to do with the diapers that Juliette asked me to buy. "Outside supplies are not allowed," she was told. Never mind that the ones provided were too large and uncomfortably pinned on each side of her abdomen.

The hospital nurses and their assistants had shown such empathy, that I expected the palliative care staff to be even more attentive and understanding of Juliette's needs: a new patient, mentally aware but with little time to live. But I haven't seen it, and neither did Corinne.

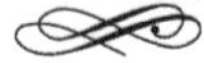

WRITING ABOUT THIS troubled me so much again that I researched what palliative care nursing entails. What I found opened my mind in more than one way and is the reason I share it, here.

I learned from the *Journal of Medical Humanities* that the seemingly guarded, detached attitude of today's nurses is the required shield against *compathy*—living the distress of a patient. Whereas it seems beneficial to the caregiving relationship, it can impair a nurse's ability to give proper care.

What I saw as indifference is a part of the palliative care

nursing protocol.

In fact, I had met a *compathetic* nurse: Nadège, the hospital head nurse. From the conversation I heard in a store, her devotion to her patients affects her family; she is physically drained and emotionally unavailable after a day's work.

Obviously, not all nurses abide by that protocol, but the new complexity of their profession is evident. The progress of biomedical technologies extends the lives of patients with conditions that require complicated care from a "prospect of longevity unimaginable in the past."

What I observed is limited to one case, in one hospital, and not meant as a generalization of the profession in Switzerland or elsewhere.

In fact, the American Nurses Association issued a significant call for action in 2017, emphasizing they 'receive less than optimal palliative and hospice care education,' and regretting a work overload that doesn't allow 'person-centered palliative care.'

Nurses and their assistants complain of overwork and underpay. This is not the case in Switzerland, where healthcare is not socialized, is expensive, and nurses are well paid.

As I would later learn through a friend who lost loved ones to pancreatic cancer, yet has a survivor in her family, had Juliette lived in the United States she could have received the compassion she needed from an organization such as, indeed, PanCAN. But, to my knowledge, such support is offered neither in Switzerland nor in France. The reason? Charitable organizations depend on donors, a mindset that seems to be less prevalent in France and Switzerland, in part because donations are not as incentively tax-deductible as they are in the United States—or

Canada. French donors respond better to the annual television marathon, known as AFM/Telethon, with non-stop entertainment over thirty hours, and raising more than eighty million euros in 2023.

PanCAN not only funds research and help patients find the latest experimental therapies, but also provides free, personalized guidance and information, emotionally supporting the patients *and* their families by helping them every step of the way. Because no one can do it alone.

In the end, the only compassion and nurturing Juliette received after I left was from Corinne, who stayed with her mother day and night. Corinne, who needed compassion, too.

As for the staff indifference, Juliette alluded to it, although not overtly, as if she was ashamed not to be worth better anymore. One day, she mentioned that a priest had an office next door. I thought she might finally accept his guidance if not his nurturing. She never did.

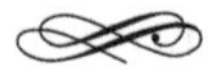

ON THAT SAME afternoon, a nurse assistant comes in, holding a medication tray. Juliette hasn't seen this person before and wants to know what the pills are for and see their packaging. She is allergic to specific chemicals, and to a pill that had to be switched for another. Her survival instincts are alive and well.

"You came at the best time," she says when we are alone again. "Thank you for all you have done." Her heart-warming appreciation appeases what has been a heart-wrenching experience. "I know it won't be long… until I become unaware… I feel more and more sleepy."

"Are you in pain right now?"

"The morphine helps, but I'm still uncomfortable. It's that pressure—" she gently circle-rubs her chest "—it keeps moving up. I wish I could fall asleep… and not wake up." It's another thing she's said before.

She complains that she can't find a comfortable propped-up position from the adjustable bed, so I reposition the pillows, and yet her belly isn't as swollen since she stopped eating. She said she would die of starvation, and in a way, it's happening.

Moments later, the door opens after a light drumming. Corinne's mother-in-law peeks in inquisitively, followed by her husband. She says that the daffodils she brought for Juliette were the only ones in bloom in her garden.

Juliette thanks her but I perceive a slight recoiling before she points to the *pâquerettes*. As if she can only connect with the wild small daisies out her window. As if their petite-ness matches the minute thread of life she is hanging on to.

Out of consideration, I want to end my visit, but Juliette wishes me to stay. Absent-mindedly, I observe rather than get into their conversation.

I'll leave in a few days and know exactly when and where to. Juliette will leave too, highjacked by cancer, but she doesn't know when, and *where* remains a mystery.

It's her last winter, and it angers me to associate everything about Juliette with the last time for *this* or *that*. It reminds me of sitting by the window in California, wondering whether my perception of nature would be magnified if I were about to leave it forever.

My mind drifts back to the *pâquerettes*, a derivative from *Pâques*—French for *Easter*. She might not live until then, but I hope they gently nudge her that Mother Nature will welcome her.

Unbeknownst to her, Juliette is teaching me to take the time to feel what I see and ponder what I feel. For one never knows when that last time will be.

CHAPTER 42

From Watch to Pearl

THE NEXT DAY, Juliette smiles when she recognizes her maroon blazer from China. I then stand at her bedside, modeling it as she would have.

"I knew it'd be perfect for you."

I miss the usual assertive edge in her voice. She caresses the silk fabric, asks me to sit down, then points to her watch.

"I don't know who to give it to." Her fingers rub the classic steel-and-gold Omega Constellation model.

"What do you mean *you don't know who to give it to*? Why not give it to Corinne?"

"Corinne never wears a watch… I would be happy if… you accepted it—"

I interrupt: "Juliette, I am very touched, but you could give it to one of your granddaughters."

"Corinne already knows about it… so unless you don't want it… I've already decided."

I appreciate her generous kindness, and since I often tend to assume what's on someone else's mind, I see a special meaning in her gift of a timepiece.

This gift that represents a loss is also the figurative way in which her time will keep going. I'll be its symbolic keeper after it will have escaped her. She knows I will think of her most mornings and evenings.

"I also want you to have my pearl pendant from China. It was my last big trip… the one I enjoyed the most. It holds special memories… good feelings. That's why I want you to have it too."

From the faint glimmer in her eyes, memories are taking her back there, to that faraway place that would be her last travel.

After she began chemotherapy, we looked at pictures of that trip; some *of* the guide, *with* the guide, or taken *by* the guide, whom she befriended through 'engaging' (I heard *seductive*) conversations. I couldn't help a teasing smile at my hunch of some fleeting romance, and her playful shrug didn't deny it. Meanwhile, I am grateful that the memory of this Chinese man sweetens her heart as she lies on her deathbed.

She then asks me to unclasp her watch and hands it to me. She notices that the band needs shortening.

"Do you like it?"

"I do, but I never thought I'd wear it." Then I cry, big tears.

"I know… you are sad. The most difficult time for you… is now… when we say goodbye… but… time will lessen your sadness." She waits while I noisily blow my runny nose, then hesitates. "I hope… that you will think of me often." Her eyes are sad and her smile compassionate as I try to pat dry the tears from my mascara.

"Could you give me the small purple case?" She points to the drawer of her nightstand. "The pearl is in it."

I undo the knot of the cordon and let the chain with the pearl pendant slide into the palm of my hand. She is pleased that I put it around my neck before she asks. Then she explains that this white baroque pearl in a pear shape is more alluring than a perfectly round and pricey one.

Discussing how to identify real from fake pearls is our way to handle our emotions, but I am not sure it's safe to perform even a tiny scratch on a pearl. "If it's plastic, it will chip," she assures me. Making conversation is as making conversation does.

Her understanding of my sadness is comforting. "It will lessen with time," she says. She knows about grief.

The afternoon is ending, and I am getting anxious. I must leave before the Geneva rush hour traffic. I look at my watch and find hers. She sees the reaction she was expecting.

"When I look at the time, I'll think of you… I'll try to make the best of it."

Her hand covering mine gets my attention. "Gifts are important," she says, looking at the diamond ring on her finger, and then rolling it back and forth between her thumb and index finger. The same ring that made her say that *Mallick was the only man who made her feel cherished.* The ring with a bittersweet significance. But Juliette chose to remember only its sweeter side.

CHAPTER 43
The Diamond Ring

OVER THE YEARS, Juliette uncovered most of Mallick's lies during their complicated love story. Still, their life together continued until the next occurrence. But after a decade or more of his quixotic tales, she'd suddenly had enough. Out of exasperation one day, she used the last argument at her disposal: her love for him was fading because he was losing her respect. It was a real blow to his pride, something she'd never said before. And with that comment, she gave him one 'last' ultimatum. Leave or marry her!

Hence the story of the diamond ring.

Their life had been theatrical in dramatic and melodramatic ways, comical too. Non-athletic Mallick not only climbed a tree to spy on Juliette, but he also leaped on the hood of her moving car to prevent her from driving away. Never mind his Mercedes parked on the 'No Parking' curb, his diplomatic license plate gave him immunity.

On that day, he had come to plead his case after she'd evicted him yet again, but her retaliations never swayed his will.

Whether he found his belongings on the landing of her second-floor apartment or later outside her house garage, it was just a matter of geography. He always knew why his bags were there, but he didn't seem to care.

Juliette's flair for suspicion always proved her right. Since Mallick never divorced, it was implicit that he'd visit his wife when she was in London or Geneva, or in India where she resided. But his lies infuriated Juliette. This was not the life she wanted, hence the eviction scenario that always unfolded in the same way.

Mallick carried his bags to his car, including trash bags filled to the rim with papers and items that had been carefully organized. He then drove to his apartment in Geneva from where he'd immediately call Juliette. She never answered the telephone, so after a day or two, he knocked on her door. If Juliette didn't open, he hollered her name, then walked around the house to peek through the windows.

These peekaboo situations amused Juliette until they exasperated her. There was no point in calling the police; it wasn't a case of domestic violence, nor was it the French *gendarmes'* job to put an end to their squabbles.

Mallick always charmed his way back into Juliette's good graces. He had as much power over her as she had over him, the kind that keeps lovers together. Besides, her passionate fury amused him immensely and made him feel younger.

But under her threat of final separation, Mallick had only one promise left: divorce and marry Juliette.

Juliette was ecstatic until no date was set, and impatience led to doubt. And to more squabbles. At a loss to back up his promise of a commitment, Mallick surprised her with an invitation to a jewelry store in downtown Geneva. That promise opened her heart again. She chose the sizeable solitaire among the rings set aside for her and refused to wear it until their wedding day. That day never came.

Mallick kept making excuses, manipulating the facts until they all came together, without being outright lies. Getting a divorce wasn't a simple formality for Mallick, something Juliette understood until she faced the fact that they'd never marry. Her resentment reached another 'point of no return.' She met such points before, but this time, their relationship was as close to ending as it ever was.

Confronted and at a loss for new pretexts, Mallick confessed.

He couldn't leave his wife. The ring was the last token of love he could give her. A token that inadvertently reflected Juliette's destiny, and fate.

For the Greeks and Romans, diamonds were the tears of the gods, but they also brought courage and bravery during battle. And in Ancient India, diamonds attracted lightning bolts yet were a protection from danger.

For Mallick, this diamond was the symbol of his eternal love, and he begged Juliette to accept it that way.

I realize I am attempting to read his mind here but, whatever the reasons for Mallick not to commit, a lack of love doesn't suit what I know of their relationship. Their affair survived for too long, and through the many complications that they brought into each other's lives. Simply, he couldn't turn his back to the filial side of his Indian life, nor could he end his devotion for Juliette. Besides, he might no longer have access to his family's wealth.

Juliette conceded, albeit resentfully, to the compassion and affection he felt for his wife. But only in light of his love for her.

And so, with the diamond ring began a new chapter of their love story.

Juliette accepted the positive side of their relationship and put up with the negative one. If not marriage, Mallick offered much of what a woman wants. He was kind, intelligent, funny, generous, and so traditionally gallant and elegant. Reportedly, he was also a good lover. She felt grounded by his presence in her home, and although theirs was not a secure relationship, Mallick always had her back in hard times.

However disillusioned, she let go of her anger and culpability. Her seductive mischievousness suited his ever-unruffled calm and convincing demeanor. They were addicted to a dynamic that let her speak her mind and kept him emotionally dependent.

CHAPTER 44
The End of a Love Story

YEARS LATER, MALLICK retired and had no official reason to stay in Geneva, but he had plans other than to move back to India.

He wrote a book that Juliette edited, and the organization published. This gave him an acceptable reason to stay in Switzerland plus the freedom to spend most of his time in France with Juliette. It also meant that his infamous 'business trips' to London and personal visits to India infuriated Juliette again. These trips, however, were no longer a reminder of the unavoidable dead end of their relationship. That dead end was coming.

Mallick was aging fast, especially mentally. Each day turned into correcting what went wrong the day before, like losing his keys, forgetting his wallet in a taxi, going to the airport on the wrong day or for the wrong time, leaving some of his belongings at the security screening, or forgetting to claim his baggage, some of these lapses happening on the same day. He was getting confused and repeated himself more than aging would suggest.

Juliette feared these were the precursors of Alzheimer's. She understood the age factor, and had they been married she would have taken care of him. But Mallick's condition was problematic in another way.

She often worried he might suffer some medical emergency—have a heart attack or, worse, die at her house. Quite apart from the personal distress, and the administrative complications, all confidentiality would be lost, the first responders recording her home as the place of the emergency.

Juliette's concerns were justified, and her mixed feelings were understandable. On the one hand, she resented that their long, alleged clandestine affair would end the way she feared, with Mallick returning to his wife while she aged alone. On the other hand, Mallick had been a reliable father figure to her children, a meaningful part of her life. She felt guilty to plan for the worst, but it was time to do what was best for both. With no alternative to have him move back voluntarily to his apartment in Geneva before his condition worsened, Juliette had to make it happen.

She called his son—she'd managed to get his phone number a long time ago—informing him of his father's serious difficulties focusing on the book she was editing, which was true. Not that it should be unexpected, but from the way Mallick's son thanked her, Juliette sensed he was aware of their relationship. How the move back to his apartment happened, I don't recall.

Juliette then began to travel, although they still saw each other, sometimes for a weekend and mostly at Mallick's insistence. Then Mallick could no longer drive and was confined to his apartment with his Indian servant, now his caretaker.

It soon became obvious that her new freedom and trips didn't compensate for his lost companionship; she missed him. They talked over the phone now and then, but he was never alone. She lamented that they soon couldn't even privately share their loneliness.

Mallick was diminished but was still the man Juliette loved and retained a great affection for. During one of our conversations, she regretted not having told him she would always cherish their crazy life together. I suggested she write instead. She did, asking Mallick not to keep the letter but destroy it instead.

He called her immediately after reading it, and they no longer cared whether someone heard them. Her written words had "brought him to tears, happy tears," he said. They laughed as he explained how he reconciled himself a long time ago to her tempestuous attacks: accepting them was the only way he could show his love; otherwise, why would he have let her treat him the way she did for so many years? These may not have been Juliette's exact words as she told me the story, but I remember her satisfied chuckling as she remembered his teasing comments.

Sometime later, Mallick informed Juliette that his son was taking him to consult a specialist in London. He would call her as soon as he'd be back in Geneva. Juliette knew he would never come back and that they may never talk again.

They had said their goodbyes through her letter, and shared their voices one last time, with affection, sadness, and peace. And when she asked whether he'd destroyed her letter, he said he would. It's my guess that he never did.

It was then Juliette's turn not to let go. With no news after a couple of weeks, worried and in denial that all ties had been tacitly cut, Juliette called Mallick's number in London, something he had always forbidden. She had obtained the London number in the same way as his son's, from the notebook in Mallick's briefcase.

The phone rang, and it was likely his wife who answered. Juliette asked to speak to Mr. Godavarthi, about the book that she was editing for him. She understood the cryptic message: "Mr. Godavarthi is not available." Juliette accepted that it was his wife's turn to hold the reins. Months later, the voice that had answered her call to London answered her daring call to India, with the same answer. And from that powerlessness came her abdication.

It may have been a year or so after Juliette retired that she received a phone call from one of Mallick's former colleagues, who had just returned from India. 'Based on their collaboration at work and on his book,' he was informing Juliette that Mr. Godavarthi passed away. A year or so before, a similar phone call had informed her that "Mr. Godavarthi was in the advanced stage of Alzheimer's."

The news of Mallick's death hit her harder than she expected.

This last phone call was also the evidence that their relationship had been common knowledge. It brought back the cautious greetings of her male colleagues. And the dash of disdain that she detected from some women wasn't in her imagination. She was grateful for this considerate last phone call that prevented the shock of learning of Mallick's death through an obituary in the organization's monthly newsletter. But she was crushed by all that her loss meant.

A relationship like theirs wouldn't have lasted unless something was real. It was the story of an irreconcilable situation between two extraordinary characters, in which admiration, mistrust, devotion, perspicacity, and deceit mingled. And in which an obsessive, lasting love had prevailed.

CHAPTER 45
The Phone Call

I DRIVE TO the clinic with a lump in my throat. This is it: my last day with Juliette. The familiar landmarks on the way remind me of the nerve-racking drive from the hospital to the clinic, less than a week ago.

My attention is on the road, but my mind wanders to the vision of a tunnel, and I struggle to reconcile the entrance to the exit. My leaving tomorrow is akin to letting Juliette enter that tunnel alone as if I hadn't fulfilled her wish that I 'accompany' her to the end of her life.

At the same time, we may already be in that tunnel. *Haven't I already tried to guide her through the darkness of the entrance, so she could find her way to the light of the exit?* I ask myself. I can't go along with her any further. She alone must go through the threshold of the 'unknown' as she called it.

"There is one more thing I need to do before you leave," Juliette says as I remove my coat.

She must call her American twin-granddaughters.

She is distraught at their silence following her emails and voice messages. I explain that they are part of a very distracted generation, but I can tell she isn't convinced. I add that gratitude is more often implied than shown sometimes. She closes her eyes with a nod, then reaches for her cell phone on the nightstand.

"I must talk to them… now."

"Give me the number and I'll dial it for you… then I'll let you talk to them." Instead, she draws her phone to her chest, wanting to do it herself.

"Please… stay… otherwise… I won't be able to… say all I want to say."

Her comment surprises me, not understanding why.

She painstakingly dials the wrong number several times, but her shaky hands make it difficult to tap the correct digits on her flip phone. She becomes more and more frustrated until, much to my consternation, and before I have time to help, she swivels to sit on the side of the bed.

She keeps dialing numbers with the obsession of someone who has gone mad, her hospital gown hanging loose on her frail ocher-colored body, her feet dangling above the floor. I support her back, stretching my arms across the bed, worried that she might collapse. It breaks my heart to see her so agitated and struggling with this last call to her granddaughters, who wouldn't recognize their grandmother if they saw her. When her call finally goes through, she gets their voicemail and begins to call their names.

"Please, please… pick up the phone… It's the last time I can talk to you… I am very sick… you know," she begs.

I can still hear her voice growling out of desperation.

Juliette hangs up and then dials another number. I am relieved when someone answers. Juliette is 'so happy' she can talk to *her*—one of the twins. She explains why she is calling. Then she doesn't stop talking.

After a while, I guess from her comment that the girl is cry-ing and has passed the telephone on to her sister. Now speaking to the other twin, Juliette repeats several times how much she loves them both. They have been very special to her because she misses their mother so much. She is sorry they—Juliette and that twin—didn't get along better, but this hasn't changed how much she loves her.

One of the twins has been a bit of a rebel, as teenagers often are, but both lived a tragedy as little girls. As the call goes on, I lose track of time, of what she says during this poignant cry of love.

Juliette eventually calms down, regaining some composure and my attention. She says she favored them in her will, as if they were her children instead of her grandchildren. She hopes they finish their studies and that their inheritance will give them a good start in life. Then she again gets entangled in her emotions, trying to leave them with some last guiding thoughts.

I try to imagine her granddaughters listening to their French grandmother's desperate plea, from so far away. The girls experienced so much loss already, and now they are about to lose her too. I wish I could help, but there is nothing I can do but be at Juliette's side.

When Juliette drops her phone, her body is shaking, yet I feel stiffness when I help her lie down. I am struck by her absent gaze and her mouth open from exhaustion. I fear this is the moment that she may die. I lay one hand on her forehead and the other on her cheek as if I were comforting a heartbroken child. Moments go by until she smiles.

"It was hard… but I did it… I wanted to talk to them… I had to… and I got them… both." Her breathing is shallow; her voice is no longer strained by anxiety but fades at the end of each word. She then stares at the ceiling and shares some of what her granddaughters said. I am grateful for their loving words. I tell her all is well now.

I choose this moment to leave, while Juliette is still in the cocoon of her granddaughters' voices. I hold my tears and try to control the twitching of my lips and chin. In a blur, I tell her how much I will miss her.

"*Au revoir, ma chérie*," (*goodbye, my darling*), she says.

It had taken me by surprise when she called me by this term of endearment a few other times in the last few days. She also addressed her granddaughters as *my darlings*. I hold her hand and lean over to kiss her forehead. Then I step away from her bed, walk to the door, and turn to her one last time before opening it.

Her smile is her last send-off.

The next day, after the airplane takes off from Geneva International Airport, I want to look at the land below to pinpoint the Swiss village where Juliette is waiting for *her* departure; instead, the steep ascent pins my back to the seat. My heart is heavy. I don't remember whether I really said goodbye, what else I said, what were my exact last words. All I know is that I didn't say *see you next time*.

CHAPTER 46

Vancouver, March 14, 2014

EVERY MORNING SINCE my return to Vancouver, I look out the window, taking in the mood of the Pacific Ocean. Some days it's gray, from the clouds that burden the sky. Other times, the white caps of waves morph into angry grins. The sunsets take on meanings too, from their familiar medley of, what else, but shades of ocher. And there are dusks when the descending darkness smothers that glowing horizon. Will Juliette make it to the first day of spring? Winter is almost over.

Every day, I expect to hear from Corinne. Much has changed and happened since we started communicating before my trip. I am accustomed to her presence in my friendship with Juliette. I look for a message as soon as I wake up, and often in the middle of my again jet-lagged nights.

Today is March 14th. It's Juliette's birthday.

Before I post a tribute on her Facebook page, I again check my emails and phone messages. Nothing. I think of her last birthday and of the odds that she'd be diagnosed with pancreatic cancer five months later. I know that her passing is imminent, a day or two, perhaps even a few hours.

I turn to God, praying that it will happen today. I ask the whole universe too, just to be sure. It would be a consolation if she completed her annual circle of life today; if her mandala unfolded on her birthday so that her spiritual energy could soar to that infinite, divine universe.

I expect a sign, something.

Before I go to bed, I check my emails again. Then I try to read. And I check one last time before turning off the lights.

Nothing.

Part of the next day goes by along with a troubling disappointment. Perhaps Juliette wanted to tease us one last time, knowing what we had in mind for her birthday. I lament her missed chance for a celebratory leave-taking, to the point that I stop checking my emails.

But when I finally do, there it is.

> *Mom left late in the evening, on her birthday, as you know, and with spring coming. She had been a magnificent warrior through suffering and loving.*
>
> *Call me tomorrow evening if you can.*
>
> *Love,*
>
> *Corinne.*

Juliette did die on her birthday. Nine days after I left. Seven days before spring. I feel an odd sense of joy, soon to be overtaken.

My friend is free from pain and the fear of the unknown, but sadness spoils that relief. She *passed*, as one says, to the other side where she no longer needs answers to her questions, but I am left with mine.

Did she see the white light? Was she conscious of the moment of letting go? Did she choose her birthday, so we would remember the day she died? I have no answers, but beyond my questions, I feel something was at work here. As if fate and destiny merged.

On the one hand, dying on her birthday was in her destiny. She may have had something to do with this, perhaps by willing it to happen when it did. On the other hand, dying of pancreatic cancer was her fate. She was at the mercy of that deceptive disease.

Dying on her birthday happened, but was it happenstance? I see it as the auspicious gift of serendipity, meeting us one last time, on her birthday, for the farewell of her earthly self.

In the middle of the night, I wake up in a sweat, the nightmare still on my mind. I witnessed predation other than cancer, that of the stiffness of the *rigor mortis* coming to imprison her body. It manifested as a draft hovering in a dark, ghostly shape.

I turn on the light and reach for the glass of water on my nightstand, quivering at the macabre thought. I think of her body deserted by life and already beginning its transformation into a bare skeleton. Like coral.

But I don't want to think of 'theories' anymore. I want the assurance of a loving, peaceful, eternal *there*. I even think it would be okay if *there* is nothing but an infinite void. An unending peace. An eternal peace.

I then post an announcement on her Facebook account: *Juliette left us today, on her birthday*. Shortly after, I feel the urge to address her, even if it's already the memory of her.

> *It's your birthday… I'd like to look into your eyes and tell you that it's going to be all right. You told me you would know before I do how it is 'there.' Through the illness and the suffering and the sadness, you always tried to keep your*

humor. I think of you with all the affection that I've had for you for so many years. So long, my dear friend…

Her French granddaughter posted a moving tribute, sharing her admiration for her grandmother, thanking her for having taught her 'how to live' and for having been 'such a marvelous *grand-mère*.' She posted a picture of herself as a baby in Juliette's arms. She even envisioned her grandmother's 'last trip as the most thrilling of all.' Juliette would have liked that.

One year ago, she posted happy birthday wishes to 'Nini.' I knew she plays the guitar and, from her subsequent posts, that she writes beautifully and sings too. Juliette had said that.

Before today, some of Juliette's friends also posted good wishes, words of support for each other, and prayers. We all hoped she would go peacefully, in her sleep. Someone she knew from hunting trips in Alsace—she didn't hunt but was invited by a friend—posted a message to ask what happened to Juliette. He was sorry for our sadness and remembered her as a pleasant, cheerful person. Daria, her next-door neighbor posted wholehearted, loving tributes, in French, such as this one meant to be from Juliette's other neighbour-friend, too:

Hello Juliette,

On your birthday, we, your friends, would like to give you a big hug—it's difficult not to go to your door, ring your doorbell, and see your beautiful smile, too sad not to be able to listen and laugh with you as you tell the stories of your life, and even harder not to share a nice little wine in your company. But wherever you are going, know that we are both here, very much thinking of you. Happy birthday, beautiful Juliette. We love you.

Daria and Yvette

Two days before Juliette died, Daria posted another Facebook message. Without news for three days, she was so sad, all she could do was pray for a gentle passing. Then, a man—she wasn't sure whether it was Juliette's son or son-in-law—called her to say that contacting or visiting Juliette was no longer permitted—she wasn't recognizing anyone anymore. Daria then walked into Juliette's garden that felt 'so empty and so sad' without her.

Her neighbors missed her, and since they were close friends, they needed to know more and couldn't let go. To be present or not at such a time is a difficult decision for friends, who must give careful thought to the circumstances.

Living next door to Juliette, Daria and her husband were in Juliette's daily life. They were caring and helpful before and after Juliette's diagnosis. Their friendship often filled the gap left by Juliette's lack of family closeness.

Corinne, however, couldn't relate to that closeness. Even when she had that opportunity, it ended up causing disappointment.

Juliette wanted her friends to have mementos to remember her by. When this didn't happen, Daria asked whether she could have her painting back, the one in Juliette's kitchen—Daria wondered whether Juliette's children even liked that painting. When this didn't happen either, Daria's husband took back their gift of a wind chime—to remember Juliette by the familiar sound at her front door. This was an unwelcome move.

As for Juliette's other neighbor, she only has her memories of Juliette. Those are likely enough, but it's not the point.

Before this happened, Corinne had been upset too.

Despite the family's wish for no more visitors, Daria's husband kept his promise of a travel mug that Juliette wanted for her birthday. I don't remember whether he came early on the day Juliette died, or on the day before, but Corinne took his visit—understandably—as an intrusion.

My journey along with Juliette's illness ended with Corinne's email. I don't shed a tear; perhaps because I refuse to let the story of our friendship end with her death.

CHAPTER 47

The Days Thereafter

IT TAKES ME a few minutes when I wake up to realize that today is the day after Juliette died. Other than her absence, the unpredictable and rapid evolution of my friend's cancer revives the muffled fear of tomorrow's uncertainty.

It's already late afternoon in France, and I am impatient to call Corinne.

"*Maman* asked for you for two days," she says.

I know Corinne didn't mean to upset me, but I am devastated. I failed my friend. I think of our last day together, of her emotional call to her granddaughters that may have blurred that I was returning home to Vancouver the next day.

"She declined rapidly during these two days, then she stopped talking." As Corinne puts the situation in perspective, I again notice that she no longer refers to Juliette as *ma mère* (*my mother)* but as *Maman* (*Mommy*). She sounds fatigued as she recounts how she spent the last six days and nights alone at her mother's side, holding her hand, cupping her cheek, kissing her forehead, and sleeping on the floor.

Corinne's newly found deep affection for her mother reminds me of what happened early on, after Juliette's surgery. Corinne wanted to hold her mother's hand, but Juliette kept withdrawing it. Corinne insisted, holding on to it until Juliette finally surrendered. It was the first of many steps toward some closeness. Their conversations would be challenging as they engaged in self-therapy, but reconciliation began at that moment.

I want to know everything about Juliette's last moments. How *it* happened.

Before going for a quick lunch with her husband and her children, Corinne whispered in her mother's ear that she'd be back shortly. When she did, after her family returned home, Juliette's breathing had changed. The nurse confirmed what Corinne already knew.

Juliette passed away shortly after.

She may have decided to glide into the 'tunnel of light' while her family was out but waited for Corinne before departing entirely from this life. As if she wanted to give her that consolation.

Corinne had prepared herself for that moment and did what she could to prepare her mother for hers. She stayed with her deceased mother for a few hours, comforted by these very thoughts.

All had been done and said as I had hoped it would.

Before we end our telephone conversation, Corinne is relieved that the unavoidable happened, but she already feels the void that her mother left.

A month later, I receive a long Facebook message from Corinne.

Hello dear Marie-Claude!

I was so happy to read your mail and to know that you

are watching the beautiful series of Eckhart Tolle with Oprah. I loved it. I am happy that you practice yoga. When we realize how beneficial it is to our well-being, we would like all the people we love to benefit from it too. It's so true that it uncovers emotions and lets new energies flow through. Then comes the practice of meditation that opens space inside of us that we didn't know we had.

I think of you often and I wish you and Jim lots of new adventures and new energies. Here things are okay, but like you, I have trouble realizing that she is gone. It seems so near and yet so far. According to Buddhism, reincarnation happens after forty-nine days. As I know her, and if it's true, she will be reborn soon. Many times, before she passed, I wished her to be reincarnated as a person who helps lots of people. Considering all the unbelievably hard work she has done before leaving, she will succeed in this.

My mommy… I will love her until the day I die, and I thank her every day for everything. In front of her framed picture in the living room, there is always a fresh flower from the garden. I cry and smile as I think of her.

Carry on your path. There is no goal; it's each step that is the journey. We'll speak on the phone soon.

Hugs and kisses,

Corinne

Corinne's poignant 'my mommy' brings me to tears. I wish Juliette could read or hear her daughter's words, know of her daughter's communion with her memory, and her gratitude too. Perhaps she does.

I am also intrigued by Corinne's wish that her mother be

reborn as someone who will help others. For my part, if she is to be reborn, I want my friend to have a happier life, in whatever way this might be.

Corinne's tucked-away love for her mother for so long shows how resentment can hijack a relationship, recklessly stealing a precious time that can never be given back. It would have been too late if Juliette had died alone, or if Corinne hadn't 'found' her mother. The thought of a garden enters my mind: love must be cultivated for its blooms and bounty to be deserved.

Corinne mentions yoga, Buddhism, and Eastern philosophies. I don't practice yoga as assiduously as she does, but I practice enough to feel the difference when I don't. When we last met, she gave me Eckhart Tolle's book *A New Earth: Awakening to Your Life's Purpose*, in French, which I had already read in English. I often refer to it when I need guidance, Tolle explaining Jesus' teachings in a new light, a sort of mind map so humans can create a better world.

In the early years of globalization, Juliette and I sometimes wondered whether globalization was the answer to a better world, as in bringing a diversity of people together, which she experienced at work. I would later expose the unintended consequences of globalization in my undergraduate dissertation in International Studies. Globalization isn't only about economics or society; it also enables the transcontinental movement of infectious diseases, among other pitfalls. Juliette and I laughed that, in our little way, we contributed to the cultural convolution of globalization.

She was French, had lived in the United States, and married a Russian raised in China. She worked in Switzerland, had

American grandchildren, and was in a long-term relationship with a Muslim Indian.

I am also French, had married a Swiss met in England, then a Canadian met in Switzerland. I moved to the United States and spent time in Spain. I relocated to Canada, and I also have American grandchildren. Many years ago, an officer at the Swiss border even raised his eyebrows at our family of five with four nationalities.

After I became a Canadian citizen, Juliette asked how I felt about having three citizenships. I still feel like I am the sum of three-thirds, without counting my attachment to the United States. And I know of the unintended consequences of that diversity, but it's another subject.

We'll never have such conversations again, but the story of our friendship continues.

It continues through the memories I share, the chats we could have had, and the new perspectives on life that her illness and her death bequeath to me.

It continues because, unbeknownst to us, my friend set me up on another journey. I know this from all I still need to think about, process, make sense of, and learn from.

I feel as if her ending is my beginning, a beginning that is rising in me. Since I must wait for what is yet to come, I keep on writing.

CHAPTER 48

Cogitating and Reminiscing

JIM AND I were still visiting our family in the San Francisco Bay Area when we decided I'd go to France sooner than planned, so this is where I flew back.

Drained by all the emotions that preceded my long flight back, the day after my return I rested on the same sofa where I'd nursed bronchitis before leaving to 'accompany' Juliette on a much different trip than mine. I looked at the same natural surroundings: the creek, the trees, the birds quenching their thirst in the fountain, and the squirrels darting up and down the redwood trees. The vibrant presence of the animals was comforting, even the cackling of the turkeys, but I never saw the limping fawn again.

For days, thoughts kept bumping into each other, even of how Juliette would have put her witty spin on the story of my unpleasant encounter with U.S. immigration at San Francisco International Airport.

Why did I depart from the U.S. to go to France and go back to the U.S. instead of going *home* to Canada? the officer had asked.

He then wanted proof of my Abandonment of Lawful Permanent Resident Status—by surrendering my 'green' card. I was confounded, having 'abandoned' it over a decade ago. With no proof, I faced deportation and although I wasn't sure whether it would be to Switzerland, France, or Canada, I couldn't let it happen. Even the sad circumstances of my trip didn't help; nor did pointing out that this proof was available in the immigration electronic system at the border—the last time I drove instead of fly from Canada to the U.S. Much to my embarrassment, the officer's reaction attracted other travelers' attention. I could argue my case in front of a judge, he said. Thankfully, a senior officer came to my rescue and advised me to always carry that proof, just in case. The U.S. was my home for seventeen years, is home to a part of our family, and I had dutifully changed my status, but none of this mattered. Tearful, I felt like an outcast when I met my son at the arrival hall.

Back in Canada, I immediately requested all my records from the U.S. Department of Homeland Security—a right under the U.S. Freedom of Information Act. I was both impressed and shocked to receive a DVD with sixty-six pages of records, including *the proof*. Expatriation has ways to remind you of it.

It has been a few months since that incident, and although Juliette's physical presence belongs to the past, I still feel her in this new present. I catch myself looking for a sign in the sky, and for some reason, I imagine a curlicue looping in the breeze, like a lock of hair.

I have been wearing the maroon blazer that Juliette gave me, each time acknowledging that it suits my hair and my complexion because Juliette said so. Her watch on my wrist reminds me to slow down because I told her so. And I will wear her pearl pendant for Easter. She would have liked all of this.

This mystifying transition reminds me of what another

friend, Renate, said when her husband died of a heart attack after shoveling snow: "We are nothing; one moment is one way, and the next can be upside down, never to be the same again." In my case, 'never to be the same again' means that my experiences with Juliette can never be anticipated again.

Juliette spent most of the winter in a hospital bed; I wonder about her garden and whether her house is sold. Thinking of here and there, of now and then, draws a melancholic sigh. I miss our animated debates that could have started with a comment, such as, "*Oh là là!* The presidential election is over. What a disaster! Let's talk!"

She often gloated over the *rocambolesque* lives of politicians as if their extraordinary and improbable dramas made hers more acceptable. Her knack for that kind of chatting was highly entertaining, and she told such stories with gusto until that enthusiasm escalated into a contagious laugh. So was the story of a presidential candidate whose wife left during his electoral campaign, returning just in time to give France an official photograph of a perfect, blended first family, before leaving again. Then, a few months later, a new 'first lady'—not an official title in France—took on the role yet with discretion and dignity. Juliette never had second thoughts about voting for him.

She was blown away that I'd met President George H.W. Bush, in a semi-private business setting. I must say it blew my mind too for I have never met a French president.

Since I like to read (and write!) true stories, and Jim likes books about inspiring men, I bought *All the Best, George Bush, My Life in Letters and Other Writings*. It's a collection of private letters from 1941 to 1998, among which are those that he exchanged with his mother when he was in the military, and still a teenager. For the time, his mother's open-mindedness was fascinating, and I told him so after we were introduced and got to chat a little. He didn't beat about the bush (excuse the pun). "Ah, you mean when she talks about sex?" His repartee was so startling that I gasped. They had been exchanging views about his sister's love life.

It was then Juliette's turn to gasp, at my gaffe during the photo session with President Bush. The photographer was about to shoot when, as the only woman of a trio, I suddenly felt the urge to move to the center, upstaging the President of the United States while embarrassment crinkled Jim's face. Without losing a beat, President Bush made everyone feel better by explaining that politicians have 'the bad habit of wanting to be in the middle of a photograph, so they don't get cropped out.' The fact that he had recognized me for my 'interesting question' earlier on had lessened my deference. His unassuming and friendly demeanor made it easy to forget protocol.

Later, Juliette revelled in telling the story of another politician and her hilarious delivery kept me hanging on every word.

A bastion of moral values, that man fathered—officially, though—five children with a woman he never married. His thereafter girlfriend became the first-known, unconventional 'first lady' at the Elysée Palace—until paparazzi exposed a helmet-clad president, leaving another woman's apartment, one day at the crack of dawn, on the back seat of a Vespa, his security agent at the helm. "Reality is better than fiction!" Juliette said, almost out of breath and bursting into a contagious throaty laugh and tears of laughter. And I laughed as much about the story as the teller.

Despite her derision, she thought that politicians' private lives shouldn't matter, 'as long as they're kept private.' Something else she knew about.

After all, her dignified diplomat/lover was a champion in *rocambolesque* actions too. His implied dignity turned his domestic failures into exhilarating stories, as were his moves to keep Juliette. I miss the good laughs from wisecracking Juliette describing, interpreting, debating, and caricaturing such matters.

But I also still wonder about her last moment, not what Corinne witnessed. Did Juliette feel as if her consciousness tumbled in the rolling waves of an ocean, ebbing and flowing until it escaped as spiritual energy? I still have most of these questions on my mind. And none of the answers.

Pondering again Corinne's words in a poem about 'a friend' who committed suicide, I wonder whether it was her younger sister's suicide that inspired her words: "Life is just a passage, and you another me." I imagine those spiritual energies mingling and separating, forever free to go, or not, where the universe is calling.

I also contemplate the dualities in life. Corinne found her mother emotionally when she was already losing her physically; Juliette took something of Corinne with her while Corinne kept something of Juliette. Another duality takes hold of my mind: *me* during Juliette's life is on the cusp of turning into *me* after her death. I need some guidance for the peace of mind I crave, yet I know I must find it in myself.

As I prepare for my next trip to France, I know I am about to embark on another journey. It's meant to be, but my thoughts remind me that what I don't know, is where it's taking me.

CHAPTER 49

Photographs and Stories

ONE DAY, MY son is asking for an old photograph—of him and the tennis star Arthur Ashe, who came to our country club for a Nike promotional event. Looking for that photograph puts me face-to-face with Juliette's smile in other photographs. It still hits me with disbelief that she is no longer with us—a consequence of not seeing her often. Then I come across other memories, each photograph bringing back a story.

In California where we had moved, Juliette and I are dressed up for lunch, she in blue and white: a floral kimono jacket over a dress; and me in black and white: a plaid blouse with a floppy bow under a pantsuit. Our hair is layered back in the iconic Farah Fawcett style of the eighties. I imagine my grandchildren considering the irreconcilable image of their grandmother with that of the young woman in the photograph.

In another photograph, we are at Grouse Mountain Resort, known as the peak of Vancouver. We pose holding Jim's arms, in the glaring snow of a sunny day and by one of the large wood sculptures depicting life in the mountains. Juliette was visiting us in Canada after one of her separations from Mallick, who would win her back shortly after her return.

Jim and Juliette got along well, although he could become

impatient with her chatting, as most men would. He had affection for her as a long-time friend with admirable resilience. She seemed to understand him better than I did sometimes, perhaps because they were the same age—thirteen years older than me.

Juliette often defended Jim when I shared some of our disagreements, yet she didn't ignore the way I felt, reminding me that nothing in a relationship is ever perfect. This too she knew well. And it now dawns on me that I gave the same advice to her daughter.

As I hold a photograph dated 1990 and taken by a boat in Sausalito—the quaint coastal town connected to San Francisco by the Golden Gate Bridge—I remember that fashion was enticing, then. It was clearly inspired by seasons and specific trends, such as the cruise lines' navy blue and white colors *de rigueur* for the fashion-conscious. Juliette wears a loose-pleated skirt in a greige color (not quite grey, not quite beige!), and is otherwise all navy blue: sweater, flat shoes, long-strapped leather saddlebag, and smoky nylons—it was gauche to go out bare legs in the U.S., then. A greige leather hairband completes her French chic. I wear a white blouse, navy blue pants, and a patterned cardigan in matching colors. Today, trends are more outlandish, in an any-style-goes type of way, everyone creating their individual style.

In photographs of Christmas in California before our move, Juliette's hair looks perfect, after likely spending too much time twisting it here, curling it there, and fluffing it to perfection. She decided to learn golf that year and bought a set of clubs during her visit, but Juliette and golf would be a short-lived association. Not of the sporty type, she practiced three times and gave up. And I ended up buying her golf clubs.

I smile at the sweater I wear in another photograph. After my first Christmas luncheon with the Blackhawk Women's Club, in 1985, I mentioned to my family that I was the only foreigner (then!) and only member without a Christmas sweater—the kind with reindeer, angels, Santa, or other such symbolic designs. Two weeks later, I unwrapped the sweater seen in the photograph, decked in a design of the jolly greens and reds of the holly bush. I loved it because it was a Christmas gift from my children, who wanted me to fit in; never mind my French accent.

As I rummage through the albums, my heart sinks at my favorite photograph of Juliette and Mallick. She is tanned and splendid in a *Vichy* summer dress—a checkered, white-and-light-blue fabric by the name of the French town where it originated. White bucket hats complete the perfect image of a glamorous couple on a summer vacation, but there was more to it than it shows.

First, it wasn't Mallick's choice that, for the first time in his life, he wore the only pair of Bermuda shorts he would ever own, in yet another muted color: slate (neither blue nor gray!). A white short-sleeved shirt and dark gray Sperry's Topsiders shoes complete his outfit and, most outrageous when one knows the man, he wears no socks. He looks both amused and bashful to find himself in such an alien attire lest someone in this little town of Brittany should recognize him. The next day, something else would grab people's attention.

Their trip coincided with the terrorist attack on the Twin Towers in New York City—on September 11, 2001. Like everyone else, Juliette and Mallick spent most of the following night glued to the television, horrified by the enormity of the tragedy. The next morning, they were sitting at an outdoor café when a group of young French Arabs walked by, raising their arms, and shouting in French, "The Americans got what they deserved." The diplomat in Mallick was about to react when Juliette ordered him to sit down and shush. Interfering with their defiance would have led to a brawl, plus an attention-grabbing headline in the local newspaper: *Indian Diplomat Attacked by Thugs!*

Another photograph draws me to Juliette's skirt that day. We were going to meet my friend Betty in Sonoma—also the name of the California wine valley that parallels the better-known Napa Valley. Juliette was still fussing with her hair when I told her skirt was too short. To this, she retorted I had become 'too American and a prude.' To this, I responded that past a certain age, short skirts are anything but elegant. Naturally, the truth was in the eyes of the beholder. For one of us to be right, the other one needed to be wrong. Or, as Eckhart Tolle explains in *A New Earth,* the ego doesn't' mind to create a wrong to be right.

And speaking of ego, protecting Juliette's image was about protecting mine. I wasn't wearing a short skirt, but the judgment of my kind and conservative American friend would reflect on *me*. Or so I thought.

Next is a photograph taken by Juliette for my fortieth birthday, with Marlene, a Swiss friend. The three of us look radiant, even though Juliette wears all black in the middle of summer. The table set in her patio is like a still-life painting: a white tablecloth in a print of yellow lemons and green leaves, and on our plates, a red tomato coulis surrounds a summer vegetable terrine. A basket of sliced baguette, a bottle of Evian, and Alsace wine in a transparent cooler complete the setting. This reminds me of the surprise party thrown by Jim and our children for my over-the-hill event, then joining the family vacation place in Port Leucate in southern France and ending the celebration in Paris with Marianne—Jean-Paul was still alive then.

A bunch of photographs is from Juliette in Spain, where we spent part of the year until our first grandchild was born. Juliette loved the guest room and its intricate lattice shutters that let you secretly peek outside—an Andalusian style rooted in eight hundred years of Moorish presence. A picture in a magazine had inspired the chest of drawers; integrated with the window seat, it's upholstered in the same quilted fabric as the headboard and bedspread: white with a geometry of stars in muted colors. Compared to the Pacific Northwest, I miss that Mediterranean warm ambiance.

From the date behind the photograph, Juliette would die ten years, one month, and ten days later... Do I keep looking? Photographs can be cruel.

Photographs of our trip to Jerez de la Frontera led to a story that Juliette told with her usual gusto.

After a ninety-minute drive from Marbella and a thirty-minute attempt at finding our hotel, Jim had lost both temper and sense of direction. Either the locals gave me confusing information, or something got lost in translation. Their dialect, though, was different from the one spoken in our Andalusian area, itself very different from Castilian Spanish—the standard language for television and radio. In my defense, their pointing in opposite directions had nothing to do with my misinterpretation: there were two opposite ways to get there.

All roads somehow led to our hotel despite the maze of narrow streets that forced a frustrated Jim to drive from dead ends, in reverse gear. An hour later, at a typical bodega with 'arches and columns,' as she noticed, Juliette recounted our eventful day, *tapas and* a few glasses of *fino*—the local fortified wine—fueling her exuberance. In typical fashion, she had done her homework about that iconic culinary Spanish custom, proving me half wrong about the origin of the *tapas*, meaning *lids*.

As the story goes, it originated in the thirteenth century when King Alfonso stopped at a coastal inn and ordered wine and ham. When a man in his entourage noticed the wind lifting the sand, he covered the king's glass with a slice of ham to protect the wine. The king liked the pairing so much that he ordered another glass with the same lid. And the rest is history.

That evening, we enjoyed a flamenco performance at a tavern of the *Casco Historico* (Historic Quarter), singers pouring their hearts out in impassionate, sometimes defiant, and howling throaty voices; dancers rhythmically stomping their feet, clapping their hands, and snapping their fingers. We took in the guitarists' mastery of the *cante jondo*, the gypsy style of the Andalusian flamenco—a UNESCO Intangible Cultural Heritage of Humanity. The musicians' powerful voices, combined with the distinctive *toque* of the guitar into percussive sounds, enthralled both the performers and the audience. Juliette bought a CD that she often played when we were together.

Photos of our visit to the Alhambra in Granada, famous for the elegant architecture and meticulous craftsmanship of the Moors, generated an animated conversation about Christians and Jews; they were free to practice their religion under Muslim rule—albeit in their quarters—until the armies of Queen Isabella reconquered southern Spain and destroyed that tolerant ethnic diversity. As a home gardener, Juliette was impressed that the lovely thirteenth-century fountains of the Palacio del Generalife were still fed by the clever irrigation network created by the Moors, bringing water from the nearby Sierra Nevada to the gardens and orchards of the community.

I then let an emotional *aww* escape at a photograph of Mallick apparently bragging over the gold paper crown on his head—in celebration of the Epiphany, the arrival of the Three Wise Men in Bethlehem. According to French tradition, whoever discovers a token in the shape of a king or queen in a slice of *galette*—a flat puff-pastry cake—then gets to wear a gold or silver crown. And since the name is *galette des rois*—meaning *kings' galette*—the queen was evidently added later. The pastry is often filled with a sweet almond paste, but my grandmother made it *brioche*-style and I still crave its strong yeasty fragrance. On the table is a tablecloth in an unusual patchwork of animal prints in tones of black, brown, and ocher—that color yet again. I am grateful for Juliette and Mallick's smiles.

Then, among other photographs, is a postcard—written in French—of the Ryōan-Ji Temple in Kyoto. I had all but forgotten about Juliette's trip to Japan.

May 10, 2010

Dear Marie-Claude and Jim,

This is the monastery where we spent one night. An interesting experience! I love my trip to Japan, especially Tokyo, beautiful and busy at night as well as during the day. What has impressed me the most, though, is Mount Fuji.

We went to see it on a beautiful sunny day: it was per-

fect and majestic. I took many photos and hope they will be okay (for once!). Lots of love to both.
Juliette

Ah, it reminds me that, unfamiliar with digital cameras, in 2001, I deleted the pictures of Mount Fuji before they had been uploaded to our laptop.

Juliette's postcard is of the sand garden at the Ryōan-Ji temple. We didn't go to Kyoto, so I looked it up: it may be the most famous rock garden in Japan, going back to Shogun times. I ponder Juliette's choice of a card depicting the serene minimalism of Zen Buddhism: individual rocks of various shapes standing on mossy islands, themselves isolated by raked gravel. I can't help noticing how the void between each island emphasizes their oneness, if not their aloneness. It may have been in a recorded workshop with Oprah and Deepak Chopra that I understood Zen as being, likely in brief, the understanding of one's reality.

A few are of Juliette with my grandchildren, whom she only met a couple of times. One is of my then-toddler grandson; despite her smile, Juliette's face is still strained by the loss of Sophie. Another is more 'recent' and brings me to tears: Juliette and my granddaughter holding cups from a children's tea set. I realize I am of the age when photographs bring on nostalgia for years that went by too fast.

A few others are of Christmas at Juliette's: Jim opening a bottle of Champagne in her kitchen—Mallick had died, then; Juliette and I standing side by side and smiling at each other next to her Christmas tree flanked by a low Lucite table; because transparent plastic 'doesn't occupy the visual space,' as she'd say.

Juliette wears a black floating skirt and a wide scoop-neck sweater. Her olive-toned skin highlights a flattering red-amber necklace—she called it *cherry amber*—and a matching lipstick reminiscent of the Guerlain Gigolo Rouge of her earlier years. Her shimmering black nylons contrast with my opaque black stockings—her shapely legs versus my sporty ones. Since I am a guest and therefore not cooking, I am dressed up: a black, now-vintage Sonia Rykiel jersey-wool pencil skirt, and a pearly white Escada sweater—a Christmas gift from Jim: a black swan embracing my waist, its head peeking above my chest. And I still have those Dona Karan suede shoes… in a 'muted' purple violet. Juliette and I seemed to favor ambiguous shades and hues rather than the more ordinary primary colors.

After finding the photograph for my son, I am in the mood to look for recent photos on my computer. I come across one at Manor, a department store in Geneva. We are trying makeup with a friendly salesperson, born in a village of the Atlas Mountains in Morocco, she said. Juliette looks dashing in white pants, and a necklace made of oversized fuchsia beads that pop against the shades of yellow and orange stripes of her loose cotton sweater. When she didn't wear black, Juliette went all out with bright colors.

"*Oh, it's so much her*!" I hear myself mumble as I come across a series of three photographs taken within seconds of one another, Juliette standing at her doorway. We were going for lunch that day, and I had come to pick her up. She wears… *the* cream white blazer over a navy blue top with white stripes; this makes me wonder whether Juliette ever wore floral prints. Her shorter hair is unusually straight. She looks surprised in the first shot, smiles in the second, and poses in the third, all three familiar expressions. These are the last photographs I took of Juliette.

Were malignant cells already preparing for their attack, like the dormant terrorist cells we hear about in the news? It would have been inconceivable that she'd die within two years.

Looking at photographs also allows me to scrutinize Juliette's home décor, that ocher color yet again attracting my attention, and reviving a more recent memory.

I was in France to visit my family, and on my way to the cemetery I felt drawn to her former home. The urge was so strong that I made the detour. Juliette's house was still for sale then.

Hesitant, I opened the small gate onto the unkempt front garden, then walked around to the backyard acting much like a trespasser. There, the rose patch had withdrawn into dormancy, but protected from the rain by the eaves, the red blooms had stiff-dried into a striking shade of ocher.

It was the color Juliette wanted for the tiles in her mother's place in Provence. The color she favored in her décor. It was the ocher color I saw on her jaundiced body.

And although the photographs remind me of this, I realize that the disturbing vision of her sick body lost its power. Happier memories made it fade away.

Observing the photographs revives in my mind her familiar, guarded smile, yet poised composure. For the first time, I notice that she often stood with her hands held halfway down her chest, slightly away from her body, her palms turned in like those of a doll, appearing both welcoming and self-protecting.

Juliette often seemed on the defensive, scrutinizing what was in front of her even when she was driving. The way she sat close to the steering wheel and leaned forward made me nervous. Of course, she argued that my arms were longer than hers, or her legs shorter than mine.

Smiling at me in these photographs is how she'd want me to remember her.

CHAPTER 50
Geneva, September 2014

As the airplane approaches Geneva from the north, I want again to locate the coastal village where I last saw Juliette, six months ago. Instead, my seat overlooks the opposite shore where forested parks screen mansions with unobstructed views of the lake. It's an odd sort of relief that Juliette is no longer at the clinic, but I have a hard time believing I won't see her.

The airplane lands with a jolt, its furious drag rattling me to the core. After much air travel over the years, I still hold my breath during these moments of uncertainty. I fear the failure of this process, that the vessel holding me might only come to a standstill after crashing into something—I would later learn from an expert that, although zero risk doesn't exist, the probability of it happening is extremely low. Still, it brings on the same level of uncertainty as the unpredictability of a terminal illness. Life too can crash to a standstill.

I finally relax when the airplane rolls on its own.

A family friend is again picking me up at the airport. She kindly acknowledges the sadness of my last visit. Driving by the hospital reminds me of the tormenting taxi-ambulance trip to the palliative care clinic. My parents are happy to see me. They hope my visit will be calmer than the last one. I hope that my dad won't fall again in the pond to save a frog.

I call Marianne the next morning. She wants to go to the cemetery and see where Juliette lived.

Two days later, it's raining when we park at Juliette's former home. Past the squeaky gate, the confused garden isn't expecting anyone. In Juliette's absence, perennial plants compete with weeds, all kept lush by the unseasonal wet weather.

In Juliette's backyard, I notice the freshly cut lawn, likely by Daria's husband or Corinne's. In the adjoining pasture, cows graze in the rain for what Juliette called 'the sake of their destiny.' One greets us with a *moo* as if asking: *What on Earth has been going on, on your side of the fence?*

It occurs to me that Juliette never alluded to the more auspicious fate of India's sacred cows. They roam city streets and nap on the highways' center dividers, their gentleness said to exemplify Hinduism.

This brings back the memory of Mallick whose name never came up in my conversations with Corinne. Perhaps we were too pressed for time or too absorbed in topics that didn't relate to him. But how incongruous that I should recall him now, the innate gentleness of cows reminding me of his acquired Hindu ways, a gentle man if not a gentleman.

Under the roofed backyard, Juliette's possessions await on garden shelves. An ashtray on the café-style table is full of cigarette butts—likely Corinne's. Everything oozes abandonment. As if things could lose their soul too.

Juliette is gone and so is her home; it's a house filled with things, now insignificant without her. Instead of a connection, I feel an emptiness. Marianne is silent, perhaps imagining Juliette here. She is not.

At the cemetery, a small crowd has gathered in front of the church. There is a funeral today.

As if Juliette planned it that way.

Past the gate, Marianne and I walk in separate alleys to locate her grave. I read the names on the headstones while raindrops drum on my umbrella. Words come to my mind until they gather into a familiar poem.

It rains in my heart
As it rains in the city.
What is this languor
That comes into my heart?
So sweet is the sound of the rain
On the ground and on the roof,
For this longing heart,
Sweet is the sound of the rain.
Tears have no reason to be
In this heart lacking heart.
Why? It's not treason.
This grief is without reason.
And it is the worst of pain
Not knowing why.
Without love or hatred
There is no way to explain
Why my heart feels such pain!

It's my translation of *Il Pleut Dans Mon Coeur* by Paul Verlaine—the nineteenth-century French poet I studied in high school literature. It was a familiar companion in my times of melancholy.

My silent recitation ends shortly before I see Juliette's name engraved on a wooden cross.

It's not the name I know her by. Her grave is not what I expected. I blame the bad weather for the trespassing weeds. Lavender in a clay pot, perhaps brought from her backyard by her son, has split in the middle, heartbroken.

It has been six months since her burial, the ground has settled, and the granite monument will be installed anytime now. I imagine Juliette's framed photograph and both her names engraved on the stone as she wished it. Her year of birth will appear too, for everyone to see, and there is a story to that too.

After she retired, Juliette joined the local club for senior citizens, most of them natives of that former agricultural village, now a sprawling commuter town for Geneva. Juliette reached out to her community for camaraderie and even joined forces with the village historian until the teamwork between retired editor and self-appointed historian came to an early end.

Most members of that club thought Juliette was too young to join, but she wouldn't reveal her age until it caught up with her. One day, the doorbell rang, and she found herself face-to-face with a gift basket. A representative of the town hall was delivering the municipality's Christmas gift to all residents aged seventy and over. Only Juliette would have the cheekiness to argue that it was likely a mistake. But, to put an end to the villager's perplexity and avoid passing on tempting free goodies, of course she accepted it.

I watch Marianne lay roses among the weeds. Then I look for the right spot for my *Dipladenia* chosen for its drought resistance, the wet weather akin to a tease from Juliette.

I still can't cry. The first time would be on my subsequent visit to France with Jim. We were sitting on the low stone wall in front of the church, his sadness finally releasing mine.

CHAPTER 51
One Thing or Another

I CALL CORINNE the next day and mention my visit to the cemetery, without further comment. I know she considers a cemetery as another materialistic concept, a place 'empty of souls.' She prefers the simple shrine she dedicates to her mother at home—pictures, wildflowers, and loving thoughts. Personally, visiting her grave is how I honour my friend's wish that I'd bring her flowers.

Corinne and I decide to have tea two days later.

I am not surprised that she is late—Juliette often complained about her daughter's lack of punctuality. I don't mind waiting; I am enjoying a sunny day at an outdoor café while Corinne is driving from a distance.

After the usual three kisses on the cheeks, she apologizes, asking whether I got her voice messages. I haven't, finding them months later, on the flip phone I use in the United States. Juliette would have said it's not easy to keep track of me.

I talk about Juliette, and Corinne talks about *Maman*.

"I am seeing a psychologist. It's helping me sort out why Maman and I clashed so much. It's so hard to accept that I found her only because I was losing her." She says this like her mother would, matter-of-factly.

I praise her for getting help.

"Like you, your mother regretted that her illness was the reason you reconciled," I say as my hand affectionately lands on her arm.

"I regret it happened too late. We wasted all that time… sticking to our opinions of each other… and now we can't get it back."

Have I not just heard that she is now aware of possessing some of her mother's traits? Ah, indeed… what irritated her about her mother was in her too. Understanding her mother has replaced blaming her.

I repeat what I told her mother: She wouldn't have regrets unless she learned from her mistakes.

She has grown into holding her mother in her heart instead of her mind. They are no longer opponents, challengers, or enemies. They are no longer on the opposite side of a torrent, its raging waters separating them.

"You were with her until the end. You have been the daughter she needed at her side. It wasn't too late for that, but it could have been."

Our conversation also relieves my guilt. Mother and daughter had needed no one else but each other. All was meant to be, even my departure before she died.

As one thing leads to another, Corinne talks about the problems in her marriage.

They worsened after her mother's death and are the reason she spent nights alone in her house. Distancing herself from her family made her aware of the negative vibes in her home. For the most part, she attributes them to her resentment toward her unemployed-artist husband.

Whether Juliette told me this or I thought of it, I don't recall, but the only unintended guidance Juliette gave to her daughter was to stay married.

Yet it's a decision, Corinne says, that she weighed. After all, unlike her father was, her husband is neither violent nor an alcoholic. Besides, she doesn't want a divorce that would tear her family apart, as her parents' divorce did. Corinne has valued her husband as a constant in her life since they were teenagers. She even admits that her temper hurt their relationship, as it did with her mother.

The glimpse that we exchange suggests that the fruit never falls far from the tree. That we talk as if we have always been friends fills some of the void that Juliette left.

When I advise Corinne to take care of herself, she says she rarely missed her yoga and meditation practice during the difficult past months. I bring up the option of moving closer to her work, perhaps into her mother's house, who worried about her time-consuming commute and the winter road conditions. But Corinne's remote home—a former farmhouse on the outskirts of a hamlet—is where she finds peace, she says.

I surprise her with a gift, a pendant in the shape of a leaf in unpolished green nephrite jade—the trademark stone of British Columbia, where I live. I know she only wears jewelry said to have beneficial properties.

For the Chinese, jade is the Jewel of Heaven, strengthening the heart and protecting past and present generations. For spiritual healers, it's the stone of calm in a storm, and the symbol of power for others, perhaps because this toughest of all stones was used to make tools in ancient times. If one stone could please Corinne, I thought jade would.

What's more, this is another example of 'one thing that led to another.' There is a story behind that gift.

On my last day with Juliette, I put a small gift bag on the table, saying it was for Corinne. We hadn't seen each other since Juliette's transfer to the clinic, and neither would we before I'd leave.

Much to my consternation, Juliette had a drastic reaction, asking why I had a gift for Corinne. I explained that since she, Juliette, gave me a pearl pendant with 'positive feelings' as a symbolic way to remember her, I wanted to give her daughter a token of my affection in memory of my friendship with her mother. I included a message with that positive thought and knew Corinne would appreciate the natural beads of this bracelet that I had bought in Italy.

Visibly upset, Juliette asked to see it. "I don't want you to give her a gift." Her glacial tone silenced me until it was my turn to ask why.

She hesitated as if not having an answer, and she had none that made sense. "This bracelet is nice on you… it's your style," she said as if she was telling a rosary, and looking at each beads: red carnelian, turquoise, agate, milky amber, and a few silver charms. I must have looked so perplexed that she tried to justify herself with different versions of that same answer.

This was not the time to upset her, so I took the gift back, planning to give it to Corinne on my next trip. Six months later, it no longer felt right; I bought the jade leaf pendant instead.

Had Juliette begrudged my budding friendship with her daughter? It would have been the first evidence of it. Besides, she seemed pleased to have us as a team.

The story ends with Corinne liking the pendant and knowing nothing about the bracelet.

On my way back to my parents after having tea with Corinne, I again think of Juliette's relationship with her mother and daughter.

I get the convoluted image of the conductor of an electrical current: Juliette receiving her mother's bitter negativity, her emotional charge igniting the irascible words that then flowed to her daughter. Since Juliette and her mother didn't get along, that struggle repeated itself with Corinne because it was in her too.

It's my second week in France, and I am seeing Corinne again, for lunch this time.

I notice the jade leaf pendant. She says she wears it every day. She loves the thought behind my gift and the contact of the unpolished jade with her skin.

She talks about nature and Buddhism, how it helped her reconcile with her chaotic adolescence, the loss of her father, and her sister later. Still, I am puzzled that one of the core teachings of Buddhism—in short, liberating human beings from suffering by practicing compassion—didn't help her relationship with her mother in the past.

Juliette, however, had one explanation for her daughter's convoluted character and it was her Slavic genes. "She is like her father was—aggressive, emotional, sensitive, passionate, poetic, and unstable," attributes that Corinne voluntarily shared in an email as her 'Russian genes.'

I don't know what Juliette would have thought about it, but I am happy that a psychologist is helping Corinne reconcile with the dramas in her life. Furthermore, not only does she feel better, but it has also deepened her understanding of her mother: she admits that she failed to identify her *mal de vivre*, the poetic

French way to say she was depressed. I too had failed to identify the depth of it.

Overall, Juliette craved family, one that she could have leaned on, and Corinne craved guidance, one that she could have trusted.

Another 'thing that led to another' was about Juliette confronting me one day.

In the spring before her diagnosis, I again shared my yearning for my grandchildren. I was flying back and forth from Vancouver to San Francisco approximately every six weeks, my visits feeling rushed and causing disruptions on both sides.

Those visits, however, lacked a meaningful impact: teach French to my grandchildren, help them relate to their multinational family history (French, Swiss, Canadian, British, American), and enjoy the little traditions that come with grandparents living close by, not to mention the continual support to the young parents.

Reasoning never helped. On the contrary, at the time, it gave me the belief of a dysfunction. After all, I wanted this for my grandchildren as much as I wanted it for myself.

I am still grateful for these trips that allowed us to bond, but it took time to accept my life without that continuity.

So, on that day, Juliette had lashed out at my 'whining' as if I'd said something unforgivable.

She had often been a vessel of good advice for me, invoking patience and perspective on challenges that required compromise and sacrifice. Her opinion mattered. This time, in her view, I was imposing my visits on my son's family; I didn't see it that way: young families are busier than ever before and need help.

I had never irritated Juliette that much and stayed silent until she asked whether she'd upset me. It was the closest I ever was from the brunt of the latent anger under her skin. I was leaving France the next day, so we left it at that until I discovered her apologetic email upon returning home to Vancouver.

Did Juliette react out of frustration, from her family's lack of closeness despite the proximity? Perhaps, but her candor made me think.

As a grandmother, my attachment to my grandchildren is like that of a secondary mother. I also wanted to give them the foundation of a future secured by the traditions and unconditional love of their elders. I realized that this way of life isn't always possible. Families often move away, which I did.

However, with time comes inevitable changes—separation due to the pandemic would be hard-lived. I cherish the memories of their younger years and especially their heartwarming question: "Nana, when are you coming back?"

Revisiting this incident of Juliette's frustration at my whining helped me accept what I couldn't change. Something Juliette experienced in many ways.

CHAPTER 52

Pondering Corinne

A MONTH OR so after we last got together in France, a message from Corinne reminded me that it had been the longest lapse of time without communication. I wondered how she and her family were doing.

> *Hello Marie-Claude,*
>
> *Excuse my long silence. All is well here. The family is finding new ways of life, and, they are positive. I hope that autumn is promising some Zen and that you are in good health. I would so much like to talk to you and hear your voice. I hope it will be soon. Hugs, I am thinking of you intensely.*
>
> *Corinne*

I enjoy her good news and appreciate her warm sentiments. Keeping in touch lessens the loss of my friend. After this message, we would connect a few more times through voicemails and Facebook, and then communication would stop.

For almost two years, I've been consumed with the drafts of this memoir. I sometimes wonder why Corinne is no longer contacting me; in retrospect, it never occurred to me that *she* may have been waiting to hear from me.

When we last met, Corinne invited me to her 'Zen home surrounded by nature,' but I lacked the time to drive to her remote hamlet, yet it was a familiar drive since it's where I went to school.

Geneva was nearer but Lycée Polyvalent Saint-Exupery in Bellegarde-sur-Valserine was the closest high school—also a boarding school—to where we lived in France, yet not for a daily commute. And so, for four schoolyears in the late sixties, a friend's father drove us there early on Monday mornings and we returned home by train at midday on Saturday. Both were scenic trips: one high up on a windy two-lane road, the other way down on train tracks and onto a bridge across the Rhône River.

Thinking of Corinne brings a bizarre association to my mind.

On the road is Fort l'Écluse, a military structure that rises from the flank of the Jura Mountain range, itself sliced by the Rhône River—which flows out of Geneva some ten kilometers (six miles) upstream.

Back to my point, and as the story goes, that deep split in the mountain range had thrilled Julius Caesar: a small number of soldiers could stop a large army! Both from Corinne's perspective and my perception, that 'split' might be a subliminal shield against what deprives her of peace—work, people, her mother…

It may be one of the reasons she didn't want to move into her mother's house.

A close-knit neighborhood isn't Corinne's idea of an enviable lifestyle: implied well-mowed lawns, greenhouse-grown seasonal flowers, Christmas lights, and perhaps a French flag on Bastille Day. Never mind a homeowner's association with imposed rules!

Her home location isn't conducive to interacting with a village community and I understand why it's important to her; I like privacy too, but as Juliette did, I also enjoy the sense of community that comes from neighbors waving or stopping by for a chat.

Corinne's need for privacy contrasted with her mother's need for conviviality, the daughter craving solitude and the mother rejecting it. For this reason, this Jewish proverb would never apply to them: *What the daughter does, the mother did.*

CHAPTER 53

Gifts that Keep on Giving

NOW AND THEN, something reminds me of Juliette. I am packing for my next trip to California when I find myself contemplating a long, translucent scarf: black and gray with ivory leaves swirling on the silk as if they are chasing each other's stems. Juliette must have thought of it as the perfect gift for an August birthday.

Passing years might turn gifts into nostalgic memories but they also keep the memory of a loved one alive. They bring up love, friendship, gratitude, and in Juliette's case, stories.

From a trip to Ireland that didn't yield a romantic encounter, or I would have heard about it, Juliette gave me another scarf. Its unusual stretchy fabric in contrasting colors is woven like a painter's strokes, applied with a knife instead of a brush. Such bold harmony could have come straight out of the color wheel—showing the perfect relationship between primary, secondary, and tertiary colors. Bursts of purple and sparks of turquoise accentuate shades and hues of greens and reds. I imagine Juliette devising it as a timely accessory from the Christmas holidays to Valentine's Day, to a cold Saint Patrick's Day, and in typical Juliette's logic, to a cool California summer evening.

The colors wouldn't suit everyone, but she knew they'd flatter green eyes and medium-blond hair. I imagine her hesitation on which scarf to buy, even explaining that green eyes occur in less than two percent of the world's population. Her chatty wavering may have tested the shop attendant's patience, but Juliette's enthusiasm likely brought back an appreciative smile.

I then notice the color of a necklace with a blown-glass heart and beads dusted in autumn shades—that ocher, again.

Drop earrings with small stones remind me that it's the type of jewelry that Corinne likes. In fact, one of my gifts to Juliette was a necklace with coin-shaped minerals, bought at an artisan show in Palm Desert, California. I never saw it on Juliette but did on Corinne, one day at the hospital. I didn't mind.

Juliette gave thoughtful gifts to Jim too. Days of shopping yielded the unusual square tray with pictures of golfers in knickers, the curiously tilted wine decanter, the quirky cork-screw, the wine thermometer in a fancy wooden box, and other enology books and bottles of wine. We appreciated each gift, knowing she put her heart and reasoning to work.

Gifts remind me of the Grimm Brothers' fairy tale, *Hansel and Gretel*—who dropped breadcrumbs to find their way back—they mark our life journey if only as memories.

CHAPTER 54

Family Matters

SUMMER HAS DIMMED the golden grass of California into a salt-and-pepper gray. The trees turned off their autumnal glow, their dry leaves falling to the ground as a salutation to the approaching winter. Soon, it will be American Thanksgiving, a traditional holiday that often brings one's family together then in-laws for Christmas a month later, and a reversal of that sequence the following year.

It saddened Juliette that her family wasn't keen on celebrating traditions, such decisions dragging on and spoiling the joy of the anticipation. On the contrary, our blended bunch likes to gather; perhaps because we live in different cities.

Our recomposed family life began when I was twenty-nine years old and intermingled five children—aged sixteen to three months (although the baby wasn't mine)—plus four cultures and two languages. This unusual situation was confusing to an outsider, and I sometimes felt like I was living someone else's life. Fortunately, Jim was older, his experience flicking a reassuring light on our path.

Decades later, our family gatherings fulfilled my early hope that our children be caring and accomplished adults. My 'God-given' mission…

Juliette and Marianne supported my vision of an unconventional yet stable family as I navigated these unforeseen waterways of my life. They helped me with insights into the impact that a stepparent has on a child's life. They knew this well.

On the positive side, Juliette was a stepparent to Dimitri's first-born son. They met for holidays in France or the United States and stayed in touch over the years. A few years before she died, she even accepted the Facebook request of Dimitri's daughter—born to his third wife. She knew it was important for this young woman to connect to her late father's other family.

On the negative side, Marianne never forgot her stepfather's belittling, the cruel words—the verbal abuse—that damaged her spirit but gave her the empathy of someone who knows about rejection. As a result, her relationship with her mother ended when she was a teenager. The pain was still raw after her mother died, Marianne even refusing to meet the half-sister she hadn't known she had. She had found acceptance in her father's second family and refused to look back.

My two friends and I agreed. Childhood is short: children deserve to feel safe and loved, whether they are our own or not. My friends trusted me in this role, which bound me to a lifelong commitment. And because stepparenting can either soothe a heart or break it, along with mothering, I embraced this demanding family matter not only as a sense of duty but also with all my heart.

Providing day-to-day care wasn't a challenge. I was busy but had help, and time to organize our family life, attend to our children's individual needs, and pursue some interests.

On the practical side, being a full-time mom was like running a family business, it takes a 'million little things.' On the emotional side, it was a three-faceted challenge that required human resources skills on a very personal level.

Firstly, I had to maintain *my* emotional wellness. Our family was my priority, but I needed to keep track of myself other than as a wife, mother, stepmother, premature step-grandmother, and the primary nurturer since Jim was often away.

The English language wasn't helping, tagging the homemaker along with the coffee and waffle makers. The French are more sensitive to the sensibly more relevant *femme au foyer* (woman at home) or *mère de famille* (mother of the family), or, what's more, *maîtresse de maison* (mistress of the house). As for the term *housewife*, it's time to retire an occupation coined in the thirteenth century, when a woman married both the man and *his* house.

Other than reading and journaling—usually after an upset—I preferred modern jazz dance to the Jane Fonda fitness workout that swept the Western world. I was then a radio announcer on non-commercial French radio: reading the news after a one-hour musical program, half of it dedicated to children (on their day off from school) and the other half to country music—for the American community in Geneva. Jim's collection of vinyl records was of great use, and his business trips to the United States yielded the latest releases. Eventually, I joined the team of the American Women's Club magazine, in Geneva—*The Courier*. We moved to the United States shortly after.

Secondly, ensuring the emotional well-being of my stepchildren didn't depend on *my* will but on *their* acceptance. In the beginning, it's like walking in the dark: tiptoeing and guessing which direction is right. It takes time for love to be accepted. It takes time for a child to finally claim that good-night kiss.

Thirdly, mothering while step-mothering and step-grandmothering was complicated. The expectations I put on myself were consuming at times. Raising someone else's children along with one's own adds layers to parenting, each child contributing its own. Failing any one of them would have been devastating, and it was always on my mind. At the same time, treating everyone equally often made *me* feel I was unfair to my son. That he had his mother whereas my stepchildren didn't have theirs often made me resist my maternal instincts—so my stepchildren wouldn't feel left out. When it overwhelmed me, I talked to the children and much to my surprise, they usually didn't know what I was talking about.

What they knew well, though, was to challenge my authority during Jim's absences. My best recourse was to remind them of his impending return. In the end, sharing such concern with them taught me that we must trust our children as much as they need to trust us. Resilience depends on honesty.

During those early years, Juliette and Marianne might not have realized how much their faith in me encouraged my altruistic mission, helped me let my heart guide me. I couldn't have done it without their support and was reminded of this from an intriguing statement by David Spiegel, Stanford University Associate Chair of the Department of Psychiatry and Behavioral Science—not Daniel Spiegel previously mentioned.

His point, in comparing what reduces stress in men and women, was that 'nurturing her relationship with her girlfriends is the best thing a wife can do for her health.' However, 'to be married to a wife is the best scenario for a man.' Often cut out of context, to be used as a heteronormative statement, may be why his lecture is no longer available as a primary source on the Internet, yet Spiegel confirms having said that. At the time, he was referring to the traditional role of a (female) wife as the nurturer, an attribute that shifted with the social acceptance and legal recognition of homosexuality. Besides, women appreciate gay men as friends for their natural nurturing ability.

By letting me vent, shed tears, and share happy times too, Juliette and Marianne helped me overcome my challenges with family matters. They backed my belief that mothering a blended family was, as Juliette would say, '*in my destiny*.'

As for Juliette's family matters, her priorities changed after her diagnosis. She rewrote her will, for example. She stopped worrying about her son, now in his fifties, kind but unreliable, talented but unable to commit.

In surprising ways, Juliette also softened her attitude toward his unemployed girlfriend. When she re-enacted her memorable monologue from her palliative care clinic bed, she referred to her as *ma chérie*—my darling. This was so alien to what I knew of their relationship that I almost gasped when I heard it. Juliette resented her influence with alcohol but valued that she kept her son working, even intermittently, and provided companionship despite his mental fragility.

Was that term of endearment to her son's girlfriend Juliette's way to make amends for their conflicts? Did she want to take with her the vision of a united family, or leave them with that learned togetherness? My guess is that it was all the above.

CHAPTER 55

Imparting Happenstances

IT HAS BEEN two years since Juliette died. As I write another posthumous birthday remembrance on Facebook, we couldn't have imagined when we met in the late seventies that something called *social media* would become her memorial too. That she is physically absent but virtually 'present' is troubling at times. However, that her Facebook account be eventually deactivated made sense.

Technology is such that it entwines our human dimension with a robotic one. Today, not only are we six millennia past the Sumerian invention of the wheel, which changed the way people interacted, but artificial intelligence exists. And in the view of the late British scientist Stephen Hawking, it's either the best or the worst thing ever to happen to humanity.

Juliette's birthdays and my visits to her grave twice a year make me revisit ever deeper the woman, our friendship, and its implications. Only perspective gives a clearer understanding, which is why a personal story cannot be written quickly.

I understand better how conflicts hindered my friend from embracing herself as a daughter, sister, wife, mother, and lover. How they brought on moods that kept grinding against each other like tectonic plates. In my presence, she could let go;

confrontation wasn't about to happen.

As for her stories, I often wondered how Juliette could be so intuitive and yet so insensitive to spiritual matters. Perhaps it's because she was dealt only hard facts throughout her life.

Many a time, happenstance as the starting point of her stories met her in unexpected and sometimes far-fetched ways, yet these stories always came together. Somehow, her knack for embellishing facts and innocent confabulations made the pieces fit together. I even gave up on raising pertinent questions.

Her vivid imagination was her creative outlet. She didn't write or read for leisure; she told stories. And she did it well. Her bemusing encounters helped her be the jovial person that her neighbor-friends couldn't imagine losing. And who I deeply miss.

With time, I stopped doubting whether I was enough of a supportive friend. Overall, I often let her take the lead during our time together, and by not asking probing questions, I never pressured her to delve into painful answers. It was enough that I listened and accepted her for who she was and what she needed at that given moment.

Bearing witness to Juliette's courage and wit often led me to revisit the thought behind my promise of a book:

My journey of our friendship [in health and illness] *could help two friends like us.*

The strength with which she lived her life would inspire women, as would the courage she needed when she was losing it, and the mistakes she acknowledged and resolved to make peace with. It would inspire women because sharing their stories is how women support and help each other heal.

Surely, Juliette would have relished parts of this book and

disagreed with others. She never offered suggestions nor demanded omissions, but had she had the opportunity, she would have had a lot more to say.

Inadvertently, I wrote this book over five years, which is also the current baseline for pancreatic cancer survival. What's more, I was prompted to begin writing it by NaNoWriMo—National Novel Writing Month—in November: Pancreatic Cancer Awareness Month. Juliette would have called these *signs*, and not synchronicity.

Writing this book has been an intense process that continues even when I am asleep yet lucid enough to rehash or deconstruct endless versions of the same sentence.

As I was yet to discover, it has been less of a journey and more of a crusade.

After completing the umpteenth 'last' edit of my manuscript, I should have felt at peace with the completion of my journey, but something was tugging at me, and wouldn't let go. As if I had missed something, or needed a *key*, but for *what*? Did it have to do with the secret—the sexual trauma—that Juliette only revealed to me days before she died? I didn't know.

Discouraged and unsure of its future, I set my manuscript aside, wondering whether I would ever get to the bottom of this mental block, ever meet the cathartic meaning that was escaping me.

I then lingered in the doldrums before happenstance… happened.

As if Juliette had guided me, I came across one quote and another shortly after, both quotes shuffling my mind like a deck of cards, each quote connecting the dots of our friendship. It's when I discovered that our differences didn't separate us as much as I thought they had; or as much as Juliette had wanted me to believe.

The first quote was in Amy Tan's book *Where the Past Begins*. In paraphrasing, we don't have a choice about forgetting one moment over another, and in fact, memory is 'annoyingly persistent' at keeping the most painful ones alive.

Despite the painful memories, Juliette lived with an apparent zest for life. Would sharing the pain of her trauma sooner have lessened its burden? She was a talker who had silenced her truth. Only her fear of death released that painful memory, likely erasing her fear of that truth too.

Still, I'll never know whether she finally told me of that trauma to explain her shortcomings, or to clear her conscience—she hadn't been truthful to me. It shadowed our long friendship because I felt she could understand me better than I could understand her, and I didn't know why.

Juliette's matter-of-fact ways had me believe she could let go of the pains, whereas doing so was always harder for me. It dawned on me that, unbeknownst to us, we shared the same latent loneliness, from the vague perception of feeling misunderstood. It doesn't matter that she misinterpreted it as physical aloneness and I as some awkward longing; both stemmed from trauma. And whether trauma is sexual, physical, or verbal, the emotional damage is deep.

And so, more than three decades since analysis had brought it up, dissected it, and named it, I retrieved the trauma I had archived. It wasn't deleted from my memory, but its reckoning through therapy took away its restraining power; unlike Juliette who *couldn't* share it with me, I *could* share it with her. What's more, when I would later share it with a few other women, who asked about the book I was writing, some released their own stories. As if they had been waiting for a trustworthy context to do this. Meanwhile, they had been coping, along with those all-too-common afflictions: anxiety, restlessness, and confusion.

This memory became the *key* I was missing. I realized that therapy had only set me partially free. I failed to follow through, to apply the lesson.

Paul Coelho explains that our perspective changes when we forgive, but if we forget, we lose the lesson. Perspective indeed helped me forgive, and although I never forgot what happened, I lost the lesson. Unconsciously, trauma was still altering my relationship with *me*, and with others too.

Understanding that Juliette's loneliness and my longing were one and the same made me revise the lesson. By doing my best to practice what I learned, I get a new sense of resilience, unexpectedly illustrated by the lotus and waterlily flowers. As serendipity would have it, I was researching aquatic flowers for our garden water feature when their similarity as much as their difference struck a chord.

Firmly rooted in the darkness of the mud, both flowers reach for the sunlight. The lotus flower, however, stands *above* the water. At night, it submerges only to emerge again in the morning, its petals opening akin to the message: *Today is a new day*.

As for the waterlily, it floats languorously *on* the water, in a *let it be* kind of way. I connect with it particularly at the end of the day, when the superfluous wish to have done something differently makes me want to go back in time.

Namaste…

The second quote that shuffled my mind crossed my path at

the Vancouver stop of Oprah Winfrey's 2019 tour, shortly after the first one did. In essence, we can finally forgive ourselves or others when we accept that the past could not have unfolded differently.

Ah, I had struggled with the original quote, from Dr. Gerald G. Jampolsky, said to have appeared on the Oprah Show, in 1990.

How can one give up the hope that the past could have been any different? But from the attentive energy in the room and Oprah's pathos, something clicked that day, as if I had heard it for the first time. I finally understood that my former perception of it was warped.

Forgiveness wasn't conditional to giving up hope *now* for what might happen in the future. As if what happened in the past wasn't enough already…

Reconciling with the past had escaped me because, again, I only considered forgiveness, and I was past that. My perception of the fact that my molester had been a prisoner of war somewhat exonerated him: in *my* mind, the fondling ritual was the result of what happened in the concentration camp that damaged *his* mind.

The other fact, that he was the husband of my mother's best friend, was equally damaging. It kept me silent until his niece and I compared notes and clarity empowered us to confront him. But the sexual offense was imprinted in our psyche, impairing our sense of trust, damaging the emotional tools we were born with.

I never obsessed with *what-if*; I had accepted that it happened, but I was unconsciously still dependent on the difference had it *not* happened.

Understanding this helped me move on from fearing or fighting that uncooperative part of myself. It gave me relief and empowerment because I could finally make sense of it. In other words, I now cut myself some slack!

I no longer let myself *feel* coerced into the infallible do-er, fix-er, and help-er to get a sense of self, from meeting unrequired expectations. I am learning to *let it be*.

At the end of the day, I am grateful even for my small accomplishments and I put in perspective what didn't go my way. Tomorrow *is* another day.

I remind myself to appreciate the *now* as a fleeting truth. When burdening thoughts loom, it won't take much to change my state of mind. I know it's time to go for a walk, enjoy my garden, read, or meditate. Or write. Connecting to *me* in my meditation 'bubble' always releases a sigh, my lips smiling into an instant of serenity.

Much to my bafflement, this also made me wonder whether Juliette worked on that too, only in her apparent dismissive way. As if she was truly a 'faster learner than me' as she once wisecracked from her deathbed.

Juliette's pragmatism was her way to accepting that each bad sequence of her life had inexorably fed the other—her parents failing her and perhaps causing her expatriation and subsequent ill-fated marriage, the tragedy and challenges tied to her children, her complicated love affair, aging alone, and the short outcome of her cancer diagnosis.

As for her secret, I reconciled with the fact that, for thirty years, she kept it as much to herself as she kept it from me. In the end, it was a gift: it helped me find the *key* I was missing. Still, I have questions.

Would our relationship have been different had Juliette been truthful many years ago? Would the shock of hearing her truth, days before she died, have been as transformative? The answer is in the enigmatic expression I imagine on her face, perhaps suggesting that it was meant to be this way.

As life unfurls toward its end, the story of our friendship shows that one must assess, then preferably accept, what happened according to our goals and dreams, and what didn't. Inspired by Jung's ideas in my *own* healing, I realize that wisdom begins when we take things as they are; only then can healing thrive.

As I keep in mind that tomorrow isn't warranted, I now acknowledge my parents' remarks about the end of life and join *in their conversation*. When I make plans that include them, my dad says, "Let me go through the winter, first." Spring is his favorite season—it's not promised, but he hopes that *his* will come again.

Nature has become my mentor; from pondering the wonder in a snowflake, faith in a spring bloom, holiness in the summer sunsets, and yes, peacefulness in the autumnal shades of that auspicious yet ominous ochre color.

In the end, the mental tug of war with finding meaning in my story was Juliette's ultimate gift. She made me delve into the intricate mandala of our friendship. She validated that no matter the kind, trauma engenders suffering that must be reckoned with, preferably sooner than later.

Our genetic makeup and past experiences make us who we are, but it's never too late to break the mold that holds us too tight. And become who we deserve to be.

This account of our friendship could have ended, here, but Juliette's end of life was to sail under the pancreatic cancer flag.

CHAPTER 56

The Tacit Bequest

WITNESSING MY FRIEND losing her life changed my view of death. Our culture doesn't want us to recognize it, and yet talking about death won't cause it to happen any more than a colonoscopy will cause colon cancer.

I got more than glimpses when Juliette forced me into her reality, but I couldn't reach its depth. I wasn't dying; she was. Still, I found enlightenment despite the heartbreak.

I witnessed how the unavoidable outcome of an incurable illness gets organically instilled in the mind even if it's not willingly accepted at first. At some point, the mind lets go and acceptance takes over.

Some of my theories, or interpretable beliefs, surged almost naturally, bringing about emotions and new perceptions untapped until then. They helped me help Juliette and I hope that those she drew from me soothed her too.

Later, pondering that death is in our collective destiny lessened the fear of it—as in carrying it collectively instead of individually. It was enlightening too that, whereas Juliette doubted the religious approach of heavenly life, she made peace with that mysterious passage: she would either meet her daughter's spiritual energy, or an 'absolute end.'

The idea of a palliative care facility terrified Juliette, yet as soon as she was there, the fear was gone. "The only thing we have to fear is fear itself," Franklin D. Roosevelt said in his First Inaugural Address, in 1933.

Did Juliette ever find complete solace? I wasn't there until the end.

That said, on the medical side, I am still grappling with the pairing of stage IV pancreatic cancer cases with chemotherapy. Despite the instances of years-long remissions, at the time of writing, chemotherapy for stage IV pancreatic cancer is questionable. Perhaps clinical trials should come first; before the patient's physical and emotional resilience wore out.

For this reason, we owe the patient the unconcealable truth and the freedom to decide on treatment, and clinical trials, or not. Again, in the United States, the PanCAN organization supports every decision every step of the way.

For the patients who prefer to let life follow its course, and their loved ones who struggle with that decision, the case of my friend Ingrid's brother gives matter to think.

He was diagnosed in July—coincidentally, as Juliette would have been, had she seen a physician before her trip to New York. And as she did, he died the following March (albeit four years later, in 2018). But unlike Juliette, he chose a different path, as per Ingrid's email.

> *(...) His tumors were growing instead of shrinking. So, his reasoning was: Why am I on chemo and feeling so terrible when it is not helping? As soon as he stopped chemo, he started to feel better. [He] played badminton three times a week. (He was the senior champion for Canada and an in-*

ternational judge for the Commonwealth Games.) He always had something going on every day. But one week before he passed away, he knew his time was up. He went to the badminton club to say it would be his last game.

A nutritionist advised a vegan diet—kinder to the digestive system. He gave up meat but not the fresh fish of the Northwest, and he treated himself to the best chocolate.

Juliette never had such pleasures again; chemotherapy made her too sick to eat, besides making her too weak to enjoy any activity.

He said goodbye via FaceTime, asking his sister for the German song their mother used to sing. He died that night, eight months after diagnosis. By giving up treatment after two months, he had an acceptable quality of life for six months, which also helped him prepare for the end. And unlike Juliette who drifted into a comatose state, he left this world aware and at peace.

To help a loved one find that peace, family and friends must be in that loved one's *conversation*, by acknowledging the truth. Imposing their opinion about further treatment, when nothing more can be done, would only add to the pain. It's heartbreaking and even paralyzing to talk about a stage IV pancreatic cancer diagnosis, but telling someone they *can beat this* is a lie and they know it.

A lie never brings peace.

As for denial, it's only the deceiving postponement of the loss. It robs everyone of ultimate times of intimacy; it deprives all involved from sharing the last guiding or soothing thoughts.

Television Hall of Famer Katie Couric—co-founder of

Stand Up to Cancer and an advocate for pancreatic cancer awareness—shared such an experience in an exclusive interview for the magazine *Prevention*, after her husband, lawyer and NBC News legal analyst Jay Monahan died of colon cancer.

In essence, she said she never had the opportunity to say goodbye because she never acknowledged what they both knew to be true. Was it to protect him? Or was it to protect herself? All she knew was that it was too painful to acknowledge that he was going to die. As a result, she never got to say what she wished she had.

No one would argue that, out of love, neither Couric nor her husband wanted to take away what they both perceived as the other one's hope of survival. In that sense, emotional communication might be easier between friends than spouses or family members.

The survival rate of stage IV pancreatic cancer is still low, but Juliette's legacy is to give hope: Science is marching on.

Nanorobots now track and deliver cancer-fighting drugs to malicious cells. In a 2015 interview on *HuffPost.com*, Jack Andraka—the 'Teen Prodigy of Pancreatic Cancer' previously mentioned—compares them to 'miniature bombs' that could even treat us before we know we are ill.

Thanks to PanCAN's Know Your Tumor® precision medicine, 'patients can live longer because they are now treated 'based on their biology, every case being different.' For this reason, 'all pancreatic cancer patients should get genetic testing for inherited mutations as soon as possible after diagnosis.'

One of the four areas of research funded by PanCAN is that of the mutation of a gene "that might be what makes pancreatic cancer the nasty thing that it is," says Dr. Jordan Berlin, Scientific and Medical Advisory Board member, targeting it 'might be huge for this illness.' He reminds us that "clinical trials help to learn what's truly effective and most importantly they provide hope, that things will come out better than the treatment before.'

We can understand such hope from such facts: from 1975 to 2014, the five-year survival rate went from two percent to only six percent. In 2023, it's twelve percent. PanCAN points out that it's 'the first time since 2017 that it has gone up one percentage point a year for two consecutive years.'

Research IS marching on.

But other than the reality of her cancer, on a personal basis, Juliette also exposed the natural yet unspoken fear of being forgotten, of not having mattered.

She said all along that dying of cancer was in her destiny. If it's true that we have some control over our destiny, then she was fated to cancer. She had no choice.

That her fate met her destiny might sound incongruous, yet it summarizes her life story, one that matters—by drawing attention not only to pancreatic cancer but also to trauma, drug addiction, suicide, palliative care, and family relationships, too.

I admit she lacked the time to feel destined for this, but she heard me: her life was worth a book. I hope to have elevated my promise of writing it by helping other women, perhaps two friends like us; and by guiding family and friends to understand how they can offer meaningful support to their loved one.

Meeting Juliette many years ago was an auspicious encounter, one that was in *my* destiny.

Since she left, she greets me every spring through the perkiness of the *pâquerette* flowers on the West Vancouver Gleneagles Golf Course, and I smile at the tranquil demeanor of ruminating cows on my walks along French pastures.

Juliette's memory continues to drift through my contemplative moments. I feel my friend's unencumbered, peaceful energy as the celebration of *her* in *me*, but I miss her storytelling.

As serendipity would have it, and after years of looking at the sky, one day I noticed a cloud feathered into a curlicue; like a lock of hair: *the sign* I imagined she'd give me.

You wouldn't have seen it. Only I did.

IN THE WAY OF A DENOUEMENT

JULIETTE'S SON DIED six months after she did, of congestive heart failure. He and his girlfriend had married. He may have felt adrift by his loss.

Juliette was laid to rest in near anonymity, the granite headstone of her grave showing her maiden name only. Why Corinne made that decision is only a guess, therefore unclear. Instead of a memorial photograph, a brass appliqué of the Virgin Mary is affixed to the headstone, her long and wavy hair a vague reminder of my friend. Yet, years later, that brass appliqué glows as a timeless reminiscence of Juliette's mysterious aura.

On my trips to France, I visit Juliette, *there*, and remember her words: "It will still be nice because you'll bring me flowers." And so, of course, I do.

Juliette's neighbors remember her as *the promise of a good time* at their community gatherings. She could entertain in several languages and with equal gusto. They miss her stories and unpredictable reactions.

The last time I was drawn to Juliette's place, toys enlivened the garden. Her house moved on as someone else's home.

Although I would eventually travel less from Vancouver to the United States, the pandemic would strike our way of life to a standstill. Change is the only sure thing.

Since then, my dad lived his last winter. The plum tree still bloomed that spring.

While writing this story, I didn't read memoirs about dying that could influence my thoughts, but I later read *The Unwinding of the Miracle* by Julie Yip-Williams, which validated my viewpoint of Juliette's ordeal, candidly debunking false hope too. Unlike me who tried in earnest to be in my friend's conversation, the author *is* that *conversation.*

As for Corinne, I will always hold her in my affection. We reconnected again—two more years after we had last met at a café; we had both waited to hear from the other. After she read my manuscript, her reaction was first *approval* and then *anger.* She felt portrayed as the bad daughter. She shared facts—unknown to me—about her mother and I shared sides of her mother that she didn't recognize. I validated her feelings and frustration and pointed to their inspiring story of reconciliation, that *she* initiated.

I am grateful for her acknowledgment of *my* truth about *her* mother, and her support for this book.

Corinne is now the matriarch, having lost her father and her sister years ago, and then her grandmother, mother, and brother, months apart. When we last spoke, she was researching the feminine lineage of her family. To flick a light on the path of the younger generation.

ACKNOWLEDGMENTS

According to an African proverb, 'it takes a village to raise a child.' The same is true for growing a book, especially a first book. Writing one is a solitary activity, yet it still needs the support and help of family, friends, fellow writers, and experts. I am grateful to them as my 'team at large.'

First, thank you to my publisher Jane Porter for believing that this story had to be shared. My deep appreciation to the Tule team for making my first publishing journey so seamless.

Thank you to the faculty of the International Writing Women's Guild, for their guidance, motivation, and knowledge, and to my international writer friends.

Thank you to my early editors, Judy Huge and Diana Sheldon, who introduced me to Track Changes and other elements of a writer's arsenal.

Thank you to Judy Thorsen, 'book club member without border,' for nurturing my vision; to Kim Arnott for telling me, "You got it." And to Ingrid Schultz for wanting the next chapter before 'the ink was dry.'

Thank you to the Pancreatic Cancer Action Network (PanCAN) for their early encouragement and partial review of a book that raises awareness about the need for an early detection method. And a cure.

A memoir is a work of storytelling and introspection, which requires tools in psychology. Thank you, psychotherapist and counselor, Mary Elizabeth Borkowski, for reviewing the book for accuracy and coherence.

Thank you to my son for his support and the reassurance that 'Juliette' and her daughter at last shine through as an inspiration. From this, I reiterate my gratitude to 'Corinne.'

At last, I thank Jim, my husband, first reader, and critique extraordinaire, for helping retain my perspective, and for giving me space for as long as I needed it.

ABOUT THE FONT

THIS BOOK WAS set in Fournier, a typeface named for Pierre-Simon Fournier (1712-68), the youngest son of a French printing family. He started out engraving woodblocks and large capitals, then moved on to fonts of type. In 1736, he began his own foundry and made several important contributions in the field of type design; he is said to have cut 147 alphabets of his own creation. Fournier is probably best remembered as the designer of St. Augustine Ordinaire, a face that served as the model for the Monotype Corporation's Fournier, which was released in 1925.

ABOUT THE AUTHOR

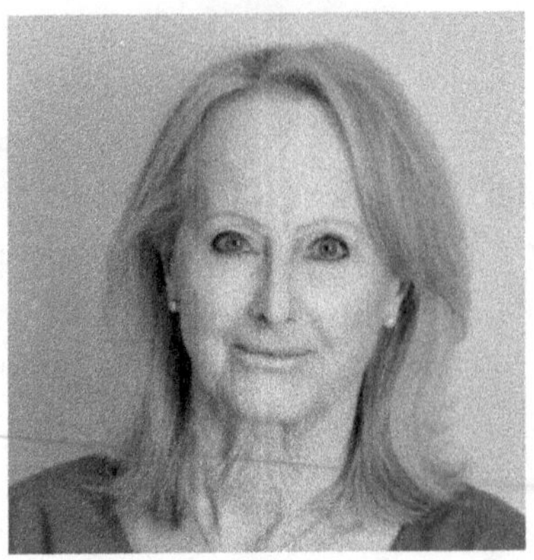

Marie-Claude Arnott is thrilled to join the Tulle Publishing Group as the first author of its new nonfiction imprint. Her memoir will be released in March 2024.

From Vancouver, where she lives with her husband, she regularly visits her family in France and California. She lived in several countries, studied foreign languages early on, and later got a degree in what else but International Studies. After a two-year distance learning course from the London School of Journalism, as per her website, she wrote for a citizen journalism site, SEO-based content, travel stories for an award-winning digital magazine, and a column for a newspaper. A collection of flash stories and a novel are in the works. Other than writing, her favorite things are golf, gardening, the sunsets of the Northwest, French pastries, and the fun of fashion.